The Virtue of Defiance and Psychiatric Engagement

International Perspectives in Philosophy and Psychiatry

Series editors: Bill (K.W.M.) Fulford, Lisa Bortolotti, Matthew Broome, Katherine Morris, John Z. Sadler, and Giovanni Stanghellini

The Virtue
of Defiance
and Psychiatric
Engagement

Nancy Nyquist Potter

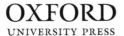
OXFORD
UNIVERSITY PRESS

UNIVERSITY PRESS

Great Clarendon Street, Oxford, OX2 6DP,
United Kingdom

Oxford University Press is a department of the University of Oxford.
It furthers the University's objective of excellence in research, scholarship,
and education by publishing worldwide. Oxford is a registered trade mark of
Oxford University Press in the UK and in certain other countries

© Oxford University Press 2016

The moral rights of the author have been asserted

Published in the United States of America by Oxford University Press
198 Madison Avenue, New York, NY 10016, United States of America

British Library Cataloguing in Publication Data

Data available

Library of Congress Control Number: 2015956500

ISBN 978–0–19–966386–6 (pbk.)

This book is dedicated to my sisters.

Acknowledgments

Writing a book is an odd experience. On the one hand, it is insular when I settle down to read articles and books or sit in front of the computer for hours; on the other hand, it is communal both in the dialogue I have with authors' works and in the degree of interdependence in creating and sustaining ideas and in putting them into words. This topic has been enormously challenging, and none of it has come easily to me. I simply could not have written this book without the many people who have helped me in developing my thoughts, suggesting reading materials, commenting on my chapters, and cheering me on as I have worked on this book. If I have failed to mention anyone, it was not intentional.

First of all, I must thank my dear friend Eileen John. While walking in Wales a few years ago, she and I talked about whether I should take on this project. Eileen's kind praise and her excitement as we discussed defiance was the deciding factor for me in going forward, and I will be ever grateful to her for shifting me from uncertainty to determination.

John Sadler believed in me, offered sage advice at every turn, and gave me trenchant, incisive, and always timely comments on my chapters. John shepherded me through this process and I am enormously grateful to him. I am indebted to Lisa Tessman, whose keen writing and thinking has informed much of the structure and grounding of this book. Lisa took the time to read carefully my use of her work and to correct or enhance it; my bumbling around in burdened virtues and flourishing would be much worse if not for her.

Allan Tasman, then Chair of the Department of Psychiatry and Behavioral Sciences at the University of Louisville, opened doors for me so that I could observe and learn from psychiatrists, health care teams, and patients over the years. Allan also talked with me about defiance and tried to steer me in right thinking about psychoanalytic concepts. Rifaat El-Mallakh has been a trail guide in psychiatry for the past ten years, providing laughter, and treats, and doing his best to educate me in psychiatric practice, biological science, and the outrages of our health care system. I am grateful for the great gift he gives me through his willingness to teach me as well as to take seriously my training in philosophical psychiatry.

I have received helpful and astute conversations, suggestions, and criticisms along the way from Robyn Bluhm, Dylan Brock, Arthur Caplan, Lorraine Code, Chris Cuomo, Marilyn Frye, Avery Kolers, Robert Kruger, John Maher,

Christian Potter, John Sadler, Deborah Spitz, Lisa Tessman, and participants at numerous conferences. Marian Potter Salmon, Christian Potter, and Katrina Potter are gifts to me every day of my life, and I am lucky to have their support. Kara Price and Mirin Asumendi were my guides through struggles along the way, and I could not have finished this book without them. My diligent and thoughtful research assistant, Mikayla Burress, worked closely with me to prepare this manuscript, and my editor at Oxford University Press, Charlotte Green, read each chapter and encouraged me throughout the writing process. Matthias Butler worked closely with me on final editing and publishing details. Finally, I am forever indebted to Robert Kimball, who provided grounding, distractions, and bike routes throughout this process, as well as daily tea service—how could anyone survive sustained thinking and writing without tea?

Contents

List of credits

Felicia Huppert and Timothy So. 2013. Flourishing across Europe: Application of a new conceptual framework for defining well-being. With permission from Social Indicators Research 110 (3):837–61.

Sadler, John. 2013. Considering the economy of DSM alternatives. In *Making the DSM-5: Concepts and Controversies*, eds. Joel Paris and James Phillips, 21–38. New York: Springer. With kind permission from Springer Science and Business Media.

Potter, Nancy Nyquist. 2000. Giving uptake. *Social Theory and Practice* 26 (3):479–508. By permission of Florida State University.

Potter, Nancy Nyquist. 2002. *How can I be trusted? A virtue theory of trust-worthiness*. Lanham, MD: Rowman-Littlefield. By permission of Florida State University.

Tessman, Lisa. 2005. *Burdened virtues: Virtue ethics for liberatory struggles*. Oxford: Oxford University Press. By permission of Oxford University Press, USA.

Introduction

i. Mapping the terrain: Psychiatry and defiance in the twenty-first century

This book embarks on a project of rehabilitating defiance, in particular for psychiatrists and the people they work with. In this section, I will explain what I mean by that statement. Although most societies occasionally regard defiant behavior as heroic, more often defiant behavior is met with suppression, punishment, or medicalization.[1] Defiance is usually deemed disruptive to society and harmful to self, and sometimes that is true. My concern, however, is for the many times and ways that psychiatrists, teachers, the courts, parents, and the public can get it wrong about how to understand defiance and the serious effects that misinterpretation and misdiagnosis can have on people. As just one example, consider Samuel Cartwright's concept of drapetomania, which he calls a disease of the mind that causes slaves to run away (Cartwright 2004). Economic and social needs propped up a conception of the Negro as psychically and physically inferior to slave-owners, and that ideology, in turn, produced a nosological category enforcing obedience and compliance when slaves "absconded" from their "rightful place" in the social order. Diagnostic categories such as this and other ones that I discuss in the Introduction illustrate a central theme of my book, which is an exploration of the conditions under which defiance might be desirable and praiseworthy. This inquiry into the possibility that defiance is sometimes good presents a challenge to psychiatry and other areas of mental health.

The history of psychiatric and psychoanalytic theories reveals an underlying value of adaptation to civil society. That is, the primary task of psychoanalysis and psychiatry—and of socialization in general—is to enable people to adjust to, and function within, the vicissitudes, challenges, and problems in living that individuals confront. Freud thought that problems of living represent a failure to adapt to social reality and that the role of psychoanalysis was to help the patient to be able to adapt. Biological psychiatry continues in this vein, being adaptationist (Freud 2005; see also Woolfolk and Murphy 2004). Defiance, in psychiatry and psychoanalysis, then, is taken to be a barrier to the adaptive qualities necessary to function in society, to be a contributing member, and to fit in with others. I acknowledge that adapting to social reality is an important value. Yet, critics of such views point to values in science and society that discourage and thwart people—and some more than others—in their attempts to challenge social, legal, and ethical norms (see Martin 2001). Marilyn Nissim-Sabat, for example, argues that racism and sexism inhere in psychiatry and that such ideological underpinnings are harmful both to patients and to psychiatry itself (Nissim-Sabat 2013; see also Fernando 2012). One of the claims for which I will argue is that it is good to defy norms of racialization and gendering that are oppressive. The broader stroke is that it sometimes is good for patients to defy psychiatric norms. This is likely to take some convincing. In order to understand defiant behavior, and to correctly interpret and appropriately respond to it, I will present a theory of defiance that attends to complex empirical, epistemological, ethical, nosological, and political challenges in our lives. I provide such a theory, tailored to the needs of psychiatrists, by traversing literature and analyses from psychiatric, philosophical, sociological, and empirical sources.

This book focuses on defiance for those living with a mental illness, or thought to be living with one. I will explore the potentially liberatory qualities of defiance as well as its constraints. On this journey, I will show ways that interpretations of defiant behavior intersect not only with our ideas about the mentally ill, but also with the disadvantaged and those living in adverse conditions. Taking as a departure point current bioethics literature on the noncompliant patient, I set out a theory of defiance that takes into account the particularities of people living with mental illnesses, people who are noncompliant, and people—in particular, children—who are aggressive or defiant. I aim to offer an account of the defiant mentally ill that is rich enough to prompt clinicians to think and act differently in the face of defiant patients or to build upon what they already do. Additionally, I analyze ways in which some people's defiant behavior is better understood as an appropriate response to their context and history than as a sign of mental disorder. Building on these ideas, I offer a theory of one of the necessary virtues that clinicians need to develop to respond appropriately to defiant behavior. That virtue, called "the virtue of giving uptake," highlights psychiatric engagement. Other insights and underpinnings of good engagement with defiant people are found throughout the book as they arise from cases, analyses, and discussions.

My framework is a version of Aristotelian virtue ethics, with modifications to Aristotle's theory that speak to twenty-first-century societies instead of the ancient polis. The readiness to be defiant I call a virtue. I will argue that being defiant at the right times, in the right ways, and for the right reasons is praiseworthy. An Aristotelian framework provides me with the language for discussing the virtue of defiance in terms of having extremes and an intermediate condition. The extremes are found in excessive defiance or in deficient defiance; both are to be avoided and the intermediate condition sought. I will explain each of these conditions or states in this book as I identify the parameters and limits of proper defiance and how the theory can assist psychiatrists in understanding and responding to various manifestations of defiant behavior. Aristotelian virtue ethics also allows me to frame defiance as a disposition of readiness—a quality of character—that requires *phronesis* or good practical reasoning. The good sort of defiance I advocate is not unconsciously driven but considered and aware.

While this book employs Aristotle's virtue ethics, it also marks a departure from Aristotle in a number of ways. Aristotle certainly would not praise defiance, as it would be considered to be disruptive to the functioning of an ancient well-ordered society. Even today, few people are praised for defiant behavior and, to my knowledge, no one writing in virtue theory has yet to claim defiance as one of the virtues. I also depart from Aristotle both in the way I frame virtues and in how I situate the aim of flourishing. Because inequalities and systemic injustices are endemic in virtually all societies, it is important to grasp the effects of barriers to egalitarian distribution of the virtues needed for good character development and the effects of structural barriers to flourishing. Inequalities and adverse living conditions also have an effect on mental health. Historian Barbara Taylor, who was a patient in Friern Mental Hospital in North London during the 1980s, writes that:

> Poverty is a psychological catastrophe. Anyone who thinks that madness is down to defective brain chemistry needs to look harder at the overwhelming correlation between economic deprivation and mental illness. Of course, there are other forms of deprivation that drive people crazy, but living in Friern I saw first hand how poverty plays hell with people's minds. (Taylor 2015, Kindle location 2179)

Taylor is certainly right about this: deprivation is materially and psychically damaging. Yet, as Arthur Kleinman points out, we should not just assume that inequalities, deprivations, and injustices necessarily produce pathological interpretations of the world or disordered behavior within it. Kleinman observes that

> severe, economic, political, and health problems create endemic feelings of hopelessness and helplessness, where demoralization and despair are responses to actual conditions of chronic deprivation and persistent loss, where powerlessness is not a cognitive distortion but an accurate mapping of one's place in an oppressive social system, and where moral, religious, and political configurations of such problems have coherence for the local population but psychiatric categories do not. (Kleinman 1988, 15)

For example, Kleinman calls the move from materially produced powerlessness and hopelessness to a diagnosis of dysthymia an example of a category fallacy[2] (Kleinman 1988, 14–15). Although I do not use that language, I make a similar case for the need for cautious and thoughtful diagnosis and treatment when clinicians and others engage with people who are defiant but whose defiance emerges out of sociopolitical and economic deprivation so as to avoid a category fallacy. However, I do not mean to imply that my theory of defiance only is relevant to the underclasses of society or that people mostly are mistakenly diagnosed with mental disorders. My position is that some mentally ill people, some of the time, are appropriately defiant, and this applies to people from advantaged classes as well as from disadvantaged ones.

Most psychiatrists and other clinicians are helpful, concerned, and constructive in their approach with their patients. Yet defiant behavior can present a particular problem and challenge for them. Even when they develop sensitive and conscientious practices toward the defiant, psychiatrists may reproduce old patterns in psychiatry that have detrimental effects on some patients. A careful and complex approach to people who seem to be defiant is needed, in part, because of the history of psychiatry; the worry is that we might downplay the ways that psychiatry as an institution has contributed to oppression and, thus, fail to recognize this as a continuing liability that is directly related to defiance. Jonathan Metzl (2009) demonstrates this point in his historical analysis of schizophrenia in the United States. One of the most egregious manifestations of using psychiatric means to contain and control those deemed defiant of and dangerous to dominant norms occurred during the 1960s rise of the Black Power movement. During this period, some psychiatrists formed a new diagnosis called "protest psychosis," a form of irrationality supposedly caused by the rhetoric and ideology of Black Power. (See Fanon 2008 for his psychoanalytic theory of Black identity and psychosis.) The symptoms of this mental disorder were delusions, hallucinations, and violent impulses in Black men toward white people (Metzl 2009, 100). That is, during the civil rights era in U.S. history, the increasing identification of unjust and discriminatory treatment by white people toward Blacks, and the vocal, visible, and vociferous demands by Blacks that white people cease and desist in their oppression and degradation of them was determined to be irrational, delusional, and demented. The diagnosis of the mental disorder of schizophrenia was a way to control the threat to white structural power presented by the Black Power movement and other defiant stands taken in demand of civil rights for all. Metzl's work raises the concern that psychiatry (perhaps without fully realizing it) was complicit in oppressing the Black people who were agitating for civil rights. One implication of his work is the idea that, while some individuals may indeed have had schizophrenia, in general the diagnosis and institutionalization of most Black people who were hospitalized for schizophrenia during this time was a way to control what might better be understood as good or appropriate defiance against oppressive norms.

We can also see connections between oppressive and damaging psychiatry in the diagnosis and treatment of gender issues. Jane Ussher, for example, (2011) argues that understanding women's distress requires that we contextualize it within the historical particularities of conventional normal female behavior and desires as well as within ways that epistemic bodies (established practices and communities of knowledge/knowers/and ways of knowing such as medicine and, in particular, psychiatry) encourage women to take part in the construction of their own illness. Norms of femininity regulate women, Ussher argues, to such a degree that, when they fail to conform to those norms, they develop "symptoms" and fall "ill" (this most likely occurs at an unconscious level). Ussher argues that a woman's presentation of distress expresses a truth about her lived experience as troubling, but that it should not be reified into pathology. But, as Ussher understands gender subordination, not only have women historically been diagnosed as mad when they deviate from prescribed gender norms that already are subordinating, but women are caught in a double bind where they cannot receive help without unconsciously being complicit in signifying their own madness. In this way, a "mental disorder" is produced that can be interpreted and addressed within the epistemic framework of psychiatry. Ussher illustrates her point with a discussion of Premenstrual Dysphoric Disorder. I suggest that an additional double bind is also at work here. When women defy norms of femininity, they run the risk that their behavior will be interpreted and diagnosed as symptomatic of mental disorder. At the same time, if they do need assistance or guidance in dealing with stressors of life and exhibit compliant behavior, they may be treated with psychotropic medications. The concern about medications is that they target the individual biological body, a treatment that misses the larger context in which women navigate an oppressive world. Furthermore, these double-binds affect women differently due to hierarchies of privilege and oppression *within* groups of women, and psychiatric responses both to socioeconomic stressors and to defiance are far harsher for women, who hold less privilege and benefits within social hierarchies.

Another historical example is found in the conceptualization of Jews as mentally and sexually depraved. Since at least medieval times, Jews were considered to be biologically and essentially mentally ill (Gilman 1985). The two illnesses claimed to be found in Jewish populations were hysteria and neurasthenia. The explanation for these untreatable brain defects included the irrational mysticism which Jews were said to practice and their increasing "cosmopolitanism" in urban areas. Religious mysticism and cosmopolitanism became linked to sexual excess, aberration, and, in particular, incestuousness. Jews, therefore, were corrupt, degenerate, and dangerous—not to mention defective for civil society (Gilman 1985). Early psychiatry thus provided a rationale for excluding Jewish populations from becoming part of privileged society. As Sander Gilman says,

> Like women, who were also making specific political demands on the privileged group at the same moment in history [the eighteenth century], Jews could be dismissed as unworthy of becoming part of the privileged group because of their aberration. Like the American slaves who were labeled as mad because they desired to escape from slavery, Jews, by acting on the promise made to them through the granting of political emancipation in the eighteenth century, proved their madness. (Gilman 1985, 162)

As these historical examples indicate, being defiant, whether one is disadvantaged or mentally ill or both, is fraught with problems. Nevertheless, I defend—and champion, even—defiance in some situations. Still, when defiance is a result of someone's mental illness, it should be responded to in a different way from the scales of praise and blame. Additionally, I recognize the genuine concern about the potentially serious repercussions to the mentally, or possibly mentally, ill, when they act defiantly—including the consequence that one may be labeled a "difficult" patient or, if not already diagnosed with a mental disorder, receiving such a diagnosis. That is, medical and cultural matrices can collide when people seem to be defiant, and healthy virtuous defiance is sometimes conflated with bad, and even mad, behavior. On the other hand, many schizophrenic patients (as an example) are noncompliant with their medications, and their sometimes defiant behavior can be seriously detrimental to them. Yet fear of punishment may keep some people from acting defiantly even if it were called for. Taylor emphasizes the power of fear to keep patients cooperative and compliant in inpatient and outpatient settings:

> The idea of doing anything that the staff didn't like was unthinkable to me—and my fearfulness was by no means untypical or unreasonable. Even at the day hospital, and even in my case, mental patients were almost powerless. We could be drugged, transferred between institutions, detained in hospital—all without our consent or even our prior knowledge. (Taylor 2015, Kindle location 4129)

Taylor's voice points to the importance of recognizing that even those with mental illnesses may be making choices about whether and when to be compliant or defiant of norms and expectations. Mental disorder may not entail global dysfunction. Each of these possibilities of how to understand defiance will be delineated.

Clarity is challenging not only because of the various considerations required in order to respond appropriately to defiant behavior, but also because defiance takes different forms in different cultures and local settings. Furthermore, presentation styles differ both individually and culturally. Dominant American culture values a more reserved expressiveness, and upholding this value sometimes results in the attribution of incorrect motives to people from other cultures or other ethnic, sexual, and religious backgrounds. For example, Laurene Finley reports that "incorrect motives have been attributed to African American expressive behavior, i.e., that the person is irrational, abrasive, aggressive, out of control, too emotional, hostile, and prone to violence" (Finley 1997, 501). Defiance, therefore, must be interpreted and responded to within the local and cultural context of different people's lives, as well as within their individual idiosyncrasies.

Defiance, as I present it, is an ethical concept. By calling defiance a virtue, I mean that it is both something worth cultivating in ourselves and worth valuing in others. As such, this book is meant to provide a basis for identifying defiance as praiseworthy, blameworthy, or neither. Many critics of virtue ethics argue that one of its primary flaws is that it does not provide a decision-procedure or algorithm for moral choices. This does seem to be Aristotle's position: he says that the exactness of our expectations needs to be adjusted according to the type of study with which we are engaged. In the study of ethics, "we shall be satisfied to indicate the truth roughly and in outline; since our subject and our premises are things that hold good usually [but not universally], we shall be satisfied to draw conclusions of the same sort" (Aristotle 2000, 1094b20) and that "our present inquiry is of this inexact sort" so "the agents themselves must consider in each case what the opportune action is" (Aristotle 2000, 1104a5). Being virtuous, then, requires that people themselves reason toward right actions, using both virtues of thought and of character, because no governing principles or rules exist that can tell us how to respond in such-and-such a situation. Yet, as Rosalind Hursthouse points out, virtue theory fares no worse than the other prevailing theories (consequentialism or Kantian deontology) and, furthermore, the fact that virtue theory is not like scientific methods is its strength, not its weakness (Hursthouse 1996). I think both lines of thought are applicable to my analysis of defiance. So much occurs in psychiatric encounters and treatment that cannot be specified in advance and so rules for responding to defiant people and patients cannot be articulated a priori. It is true that I do not show how defiance applies to all diagnoses and under the many individuated circumstances. I have undoubtedly left many questions unanswered. For example, I have not included a discussion of defiance as it is seen in people with substance abuse problems. I omitted that topic because my training and experience of substance abusers is that it is very difficult to determine whether or not the person has an underlying mental disorder while he or she is actively misusing or abusing drugs. This confounding factor muddies the terrain for interpreting defiant behavior, since making such determinations is important in knowing how to respond. Instead of sorting out the complex issues of defiant substance abusers in this book, I encourage readers to apply my theory to substance abuse and other areas in psychiatry. I see Aristotle's methodology as an invitation for psychiatrists and other practitioners to expand on this theory, filling it out in local and specific ways and adding insights through practice that extend and refine my work.

Critics of my book may argue that it will satisfy neither psychiatrists nor philosophers. For one thing, it might be said that I do not provide enough cases or diagnoses of different sorts to be persuasive to psychiatrists. For example, psychiatrists, too, are defiant sometimes: some refuse to diagnose, some work with social causes of mental distress and resist medicalizing or pathologizing people, and some opt out of academic medicine, or hospital and clinic practice, and go instead into private practice where more freedoms exist. I have elected not to write a chapter on this important topic because I want the focus of this book to provide a transformative vision and particular tools for psychiatrists, but liberatory psychiatrists may find that choice to be a shortcoming. On the philosophical side, I expect criticism as well. This book does not fully develop a theory of defiance or of giving uptake, thus disappointing philosophers. Admittedly, I do not present a full philosophical theory of defiance or of uptake. I say enough about each so that I can work with these concepts for clinical audiences. Some of these issues are just in the nature of interdisciplinary writing—it requires that the author incorporate, shift, and integrate different disciplines, and choices must be made about how much to say, and in what way, in order to reach as wide an audience as possible without being unrealistic about what can be accomplished. But, additionally, this book is explicitly political in its deployment of defiance as a virtue particularly of the disadvantaged and those living with adverse conditions. I realize it will not appeal to all psychiatrists, but I also suspect that many people working in health care services—and the people they encounter—will find resonances with the ideas in this book.

ii. **The context for this book**

Very little, if anything, has been written on this position—and, to my knowledge, nothing has been written on defiance as a virtue for psychiatric patients. The concept of defiance is unclear and confusing both in its conceptualization and in its moral status as praiseworthy or blameworthy. Historically, we find that acts of defiance are sometimes lauded as heroic, although the meaning of "heroism" and what constitutes a hero varies from culture to culture. Recall Socrates, who defied Greek expectations of scholarly teaching when he refused to stop "corrupting the youth." One might defy a policy, as seen with athletes who are not supposed to use performance-enhancing drugs but do so anyway. In this case, being defiant seems neither heroic nor praiseworthy—it just seems opportunistic. Abraham's Sarah of the *Old Testament* scriptures defied the odds of getting pregnant in her old age by conceiving their son Isaac. But her act of conception is not praiseworthy because it was not within her power to reverse her sterility, and typically we should not be praised for things outside our control. "Defying the odds" here is metaphorical. These examples of actions that could be called "defiant" raise questions about the content and application of the concept of defiance and, while I do not set out necessary and sufficient conditions for defiance, I do address many of the questions that emerge when trying to be clear about the concept.

For example, take the relation of resistant behavior to defiant behavior. Resistance and defiance may be closely related, and they are sometimes conflated to be the same phenomenon, but I argue for defiance being significantly different enough to merit a book in its own right. Howard Caygill seems to situate resistance as a subset of defiance, as when he states that "the practice of resistance contributes to the formation of resistant identities, exemplary resistants, who inhabit and foster a broader culture of defiance" (Caygill 2013, 11–12). On the other hand, Caygill's account of resistance suggests that defiance is a character trait that develops when enough provocation occurs to create an environment for it (Caygill 2013, 4). He characterizes movements such as the Chiapas' stand against the North America Free Trade Agreement, the practice of Satyagraha, and the Black Panthers as resistance movements that "*provoke* liberation, that are defiant, but that do not promise to deliver it" (Caygill 2013, 128; emphasis in original). Yet, overall, his book, which purports to offer *A Philosophy of Defiance* (the subtitle of the book), barely mentions the concept.

More plausible is that defiance in individuals gives rise to resistance movements. Nechama Tec provides a detailed history of the Jews who hid in the Nalibocka Forest during the Nazi occupation of Belarus and Poland (Tec

2009). While these 1,200 people lived in an organized and developed fashion, with guards and fighters who killed Germans when necessary to their survival, they did not begin as a resistance movement. Tuvia Bielski, who by all accounts was the leader of this forest community of refugees, first acted in self-preservation by refusing to submit to Nazi Germany's plans to annihilate Jews. He and his brother Zus determined to flee: "Under the cover of darkness the brothers disappeared. Before they parted, each vowed never to let themselves be caught by the enemy. This decision contained no special plans, no specific steps, but it was firm" (Tec 2009, 34). Others, too, had "a general desire to act," a refusal to submit, but "had no specific plans" (Tec 2009, 38). Defiance, then, even in these very dangerous circumstances, seemed to be the motivator for running away from Jewish ghettos and joining the Bielski otriad (Tec 2009, 73). But as the group of forest dwellers grew, it required organization as it prepared to fight with arms. Thus, it developed from individual acts of defiance into a resistance movement. My book aims to make clear what defiance is and how it is different from resistance and other related concepts.

iii. **Chapter outline**

Chapter 1 lays the groundwork for the subject of defiance by looking generally at background assumptions embedded in concepts such as compliance and noncompliance. I begin by setting out key legal and ethical concepts in biomedical ethics and suggest how such concepts, as well as theories of compliance, noncompliance, reactance, and psychoanalytic resistance, are drawn upon to explain why patients sometimes reject clinicians' recommendations for medications and other treatment interventions. I argue that biomedical concepts and theories are normative and that any understanding of people's behavior in relation to the medical world requires a deep understanding of norms and the work they do in shaping and structuring people's everyday lives. The analysis in this chapter paves the way for me to focus on people's defiant behavior.

Chapters 2 and 3 develop my theory of defiance and situate it in a loosely Aristotelian framework. I note differences between defiance and other related concepts, such as civil disobedience and resistance movements, and provide general characteristics of defiance and of flourishing. These chapters make clear that the project of this book is political in that its core concept, defiance, is argued to be sometimes praiseworthy—in particular, in contexts of oppression. I offer several examples of defiance in order to illustrate the domain and scope of defiance as a virtue. Then, I examine the relationship between defiance and flourishing by analyzing three cases: Henry, who is diagnosed with schizophrenia but rejects that diagnosis; Marie, who is severely depressed and refuses to participate in group activities in hospital; and Rachel, who receives a diagnosis of Borderline Personality Disorder and is enraged at the process by which she receives it. By examining these cases, I am able to unpack some of the epistemic and ontological assumptions that undergird both our naïve ideas about flourishing and a more informed theory. To do this, I bring in the work of Lisa Tessman on what she calls "burdened virtues": those character traits that can be identified as virtues but nevertheless fail to contribute to flourishing. I explain how and when virtue traits are separated from flourishing and apply this framework to psychiatric cases.

In Chapter 4, the focus is on children's aggressive behavior that sometimes yields a diagnosis of Oppositional Defiant Disorder (ODD) or Conduct Disorder (CD). I argue that the distinctions drawn among types of aggression do not yield a construct or model that is clear. I suggest that the norms that determine harms and violations worth meriting the characterization of aggressive behavior need to be articulated and critiqued. Additionally, I complicate the often simplistic distinctions drawn between genders in these discussions by examining the matrix of raced, gendered, and classed intersections in the interpretation and reproduction of norms for behavior. By taking up these issues, I call attention to the challenges that many teachers and clinicians face when interpreting children's behavior as defiant, aggressive, and worthy of intervention.

The question I examine in Chapter 5 is what qualities or characteristics would make defiant behavior wrong and why. I first raise questions about defiance by looking at the signs and symptoms of Antisocial Personality Disorder (ASPD) as they appear in Christian Gerhartsreiter, a man who claims to be a relative of the Rockefeller family. For instance, I consider what can be said in defense of a psychiatric diagnosis of ASPD when someone claims to find social, moral, and legal norms to be oppressive; I argue that it is not enough to think that the cornerstone of the ASPD classification is an understanding of harm. I then relate questions about the diagnosis of ASPD by considering qualities and characteristics that defiance as a virtue holds. I propose an account of some of the features of practical reasoning that will assist readers in distinguishing between good and bad defiance. I contrast the behavior of Gerhartsreiter with that of Henry from Chapter 3. The theory of defiance as a virtue developed in my book thus far will be filled out in this chapter in a way that clarifies what is wrong with antisocial behavior, identifies constraints on counting defiance of the mentally ill as a virtue, and indicates what defiance as a virtue would look like. The main work of this chapter is to set out norms for evaluating good enough practical reasoning for patients so that clinicians can identify good and bad defiance or defiance that is neither blameworthy nor praiseworthy.

In the final chapter, I address the question of what psychiatrists can and should do with the analyses presented in this book. I consider questions of what it means to see and be seen, to listen and be listened to, to know and be known, and how we learn our ways of seeing, listening, and knowing. Additionally, I ask why well-meaning, even enlightened, people fail to see that their ways of seeing and treating people, and of constructing persons as Other, can undermine the best of intentions and sometimes do harm.[3] Chapter 6 addresses those questions by bringing together ethical and epistemological issues that provide some direction in responding to patients' and other people's defiant behavior. First, I introduce the virtue of giving uptake properly, and I argue that psychiatrists should cultivate a disposition to give uptake to defiant patients. I also consider patterns of ignorance and not-knowing that can be hindrances to giving uptake properly. I work through a case to illustrate these impediments. Additionally, I offer a hypothetical case that indicates how giving uptake to a defiant patient would look in a more idealized version. I conclude by drawing together some threads of the book.

Family resemblances: Compliance, the right to refuse treatment, noncompliance, resistance, reactance, and defiance

Chapter 1 lays the groundwork for the subject of defiance by looking more generally at background assumptions embedded in concepts such as compliance and noncompliance. I begin by setting out key legal and ethical concepts in biomedical ethics with the aim of illustrating, through two types of cases, not only how the right to refuse treatment, but also theories of compliance, noncompliance, reactance, and psychoanalytic resistance, are drawn upon to explain why patients sometimes reject clinicians' recommendations for medications and other treatment interventions. This discussion will pave the way for future chapters in which I focus on patients' defiant behavior in clinical encounters. Each of these concepts is drawn upon in practice, and may seem clear-cut, but in fact the boundaries between them are fuzzy, not firm. Thus, I suggest we think of them in terms of what Wittgenstein calls "family resemblances" (2009).

Family resemblances are concepts that, like members of a family, have enough properties or characteristics in common to group them together, yet are somewhat separate in their own right too (Wittgenstein 2009, 36, section 67). He discusses this idea in terms of "games." After presenting the varieties of properties and activities of "games," he says that what we discover is "a complicated network of similarities overlapping and criss-crossing: similarities in the large and in the small" (Wittgenstein 2009, 36, section 66). Nevertheless, we know what is meant when people talk about "games" even with a wide variety of kinds and characteristics. An understanding of "games" does not require that we identify necessary and sufficient conditions of them and, furthermore, it is not possible to do so. But there is such a thing as "games."

Wittgenstein imagines his interlocutor asking with skepticism "But is a blurred concept a concept at all?" to which he replies "Is a photograph that is not sharp a picture of a person at all? Is it even always an advantage to replace a picture that is not sharp by one that is? Isn't one that isn't sharp often just what we need?" (Wittgenstein 2009, 38, section 71). His point is that although we can draw boundaries for analytic purposes, we can use a concept in practice without doing so (Wittgenstein 2009, 37, section 69).

I have opened this chapter with the idea of family resemblances because I want to alert readers to what can be expected, here and in the chapters to follow. As we will see when the discussion hones in on defiance, that concept too has fuzzy boundaries (i.e., how is it related to, but different from, civil disobedience, political resistance, and so on?). My aim, of course, is to clarify, not to engage in hand-waving. I do think we need to—and can—achieve clarity on what defiance is, with respect to psychiatric patients, and why and when it is good. But it is useful for readers to know at the outset that the more deeply I analyze various concepts in practice, the messier they seem to get.

1.1 Medical compliance: What is it and why is it desirable?

The Oxford English Dictionary defines "compliance" as "acting in accordance with, or the yielding to a desire, request, condition, direction, etc.; a consenting to act in conformity with; an acceding to; practical assent" (quoted in Aronson 2007, 383). It comes from the Latin *complire* and means "to fulfill a promise." Roughly speaking, compliance in the medical domain refers to patients' willingness and agreement to take their medications as prescribed and, in general, to follow doctors' orders and the agreement the patients have made. The root of compliance, therefore, emphasizes the authority of doctors to determine treatment and the expectation that patients will agree to their recommendations. Patients who do not do so are thought to have broken an implicit (or explicit) agreement to follow doctors' orders. The value of compliance gives rise to the often implicit conceptualization of "the good patient": she is one who comes to agree with the physician's recommendations and then follows them. Patients, too, are active (usually implicitly) in keeping the value of compliant behavior alive, by performing the "good patient role." Even doctors, when they become patients, adopt this demeanor and presentation. For example, Carlos questions the good patient role, but he nevertheless finds himself in that role:

> The health professional who catheterised me after my recent appendectomy used the anaesthetic gel simply as lubricant, without waiting for the anaesthetic to take effect. Neither I nor my wife, who is also a doctor, openly questioned the neglect of this simple precaution, which converted an unpleasant procedure into an unnecessarily painful one. Why did we let that happen? Did we think that being passive

and compliant made me a good patient? Or were we just too afraid to question the authority of our caregiver? (Jadad et al. 2003, 1)

This understanding of patients' responsibility to be compliant has come under criticism in recent years. Kleinsinger notes that "As shared decision making has become a standard of practice since the 1990s, we can now see compliance as referring to the mutually negotiated physician–patient agreement or contract, which rehabilitates the term from its previous negative associations" (Kleinsinger 2010, 55). But as McCarthy et al. say, definitions are not rigorous enough to allow for empirical research reliably (2010, 244). What we can say, from a literature review, is that, operationally, patients' voices are not taken into account when trying to secure compliance (McCarthy et al. 2010, 244).

As I will show in Section 1.6.2, expectations of compliance sometimes are challenged when cultural clashes occur, in part because the patients' different ontological and moral world-views are overlooked or misunderstood. The imperative to understand patients' behavior and needs in their local and cultural lives is a theme throughout this book, even while I hold that the value of respecting the beliefs, norms, and practices of other cultures does not imply or require a relativist stance. Additionally, the expectation of compliance, or the "good patient role," is complicated by mental illness. When patients are deemed incompetent, whether by their ignorance about Western medicine and culture or by mental illness, then the "best interests" standard is appealed to in deciding treatment for the patient. But the "best interests" standard permits physicians to persuade patients and their loved ones to the point that persuasion can look a lot like coercion.

To coerce someone is to arrange choices and options such that the most attractive alternative is the one you want her to make (Frye 1983). This way of understanding coercion cuts through the notion prevalent in American ideology that, as long as we are able to choose between available options, we are free and our liberty and autonomy are preserved. Coercion does not deny that, in a very narrow sense of the term, a person's agency is retained, but it entails that "choice" is so constrained that it cannot be said to be free. For example, when the physician believes that the patient is failing to grasp the seriousness of her situation and therefore must intervene in what is the patient's best interest, the physician's authority combined with the patient's belief that she must adopt the good patient role may transform a conversation involving persuasion into one of coercion. A patient's feeling of being coerced may result in noncompliance—that is, an apparent consent with covert refusal (see Section 1.4) I am not suggesting that coercion is always morally wrong; it may be justified (as it surely is when raising children). Coercion is also not purely an individual behavior. It is often supported and even backed by institutional sanctions and ideologies, as in the pressure on pregnant teenagers not to get abortions but, instead, to keep and raise their babies themselves, often postponing education and entrance into the workforce indefinitely. But coercion is a morally complex practice. Thus, I will return to this concept throughout the book, as I examine compliance, defiance, norms for behavior, and interventions.

It may seem odd to allude to concepts from political theory such as coercion and civil disobedience when talking about noncompliant patients. I hope to motivate these relations between psychiatric patient care and political theory as the book unfolds. But, as I say, freedom from coercion and the right to exercise one's voice are connecting links between noncompliance and more overtly political ideas. For example, evidence shows that patients, including psychiatric patients, do want to be involved in decision-making about their own treatments (see Farrelly et al. 2015; Hamann, Leucht, and Kissing 2003, 405). So, how we think about the doctor–patient relationship is an issue about having a voice, which is a concept central to democratic practices. To have a voice means, briefly, to express one's needs, values, experiences, and world-view with the reasonable expectation that others will give you uptake. These claims are developed in Chapter 6. Yet, when shared decision-making involves patients who have mental illnesses, research shows that "while there was a rhetorical commitment to egalitarian models of interactions, many took decisions or withheld information that they felt would hinder their preferred option" (Farrelly et al. 2015, 2). As Martha Nussbaum argues, people with mental difficulties are not included in considerations of the basic structures of institutions, either as full participants or as reciprocating citizens (Nussbaum 2007). Correcting this neglect is a matter of social justice, including for patients with mental disorders and mental disabilities. By this I mean that to neglect or repress voices of certain groups, such as psychiatric patients or refugee patients, is to treat them as if they a priori were not potential knowers about their own situation, needs, and experiences. To exclude some people from participating in essential community functions, such as the production of knowledge, is unfair unless the grounds for exclusion are morally justified. (An example of what is considered morally justifiable exclusion is the U.S. and British law that convicted felons are excluded from voting.) Yet the desire and value of having a voice in psychiatric treatment varies from culture to culture, and from individual to individual, and it is important to realize that the fairly new push toward patient participation in treatment plans, medications, and so on should not be assumed to be shared universally (Tse, Tang, and Kan Dip Cert 2015).

Nevertheless, the desire for autonomy and a sense of agency is considered by most people to be one of the qualities that makes life worth living (cf. Williams 1973). This includes the desire to exercise agency in locally and culturally inflected ways. The cluster of concepts I am examining—compliance, noncompliance, and defiance—points to a tension that is described by Dostoevsky:

> There is one case [one only] when man may purposely, consciously, desire what is injurious to himself, what is stupid, very stupid—simply in order *to have the right* to desire for himself even what is very stupid and *not to be bound by an obligation* to desire only what is rational. (Dostoevsky 1960, 26; emphasis added)

Dostoevsky is right that the exercise of our freedom is such a great good that we sometimes are willing to risk backlash and judgments of non-normalcy when we choose it despite great risks. But I suggest that he is somewhat wrong—that we are not always irrational and foolish when we act against what looks from the physician's perspective, to be in our best interests. I argue that being defiant can be a virtue and, like other virtues, is a necessary condition for living a relatively flourishing life (see Chapter 3 for a discussion of what I mean by "flourishing"). To accomplish this, I also discuss noncompliance in the cultural and social sense.

The point is that "compliance" is a term laden with value. Because it is sometimes brought about through interventions, such as persuasion, that are authoritarian (Frosch et al. 2012), or coercion or even force, compliance is criticized as being paternalistic (Vuckovich 2010). For instance, situations arise when, due to the patient's apparently clouded judgment or presence of a mental illness, the patient does not seem to be in the best position to decide not to be compliant. In such cases, the physician may be (or may take himself to be) legally and morally obligated to act in loco parentis. Patients are restrained by medical or by physical means, for example, when they present a danger to others by making threats or getting too close to others. But that right and duty to protect patients from themselves and others is also contested, especially concerning questions about the patients' capacity to look after themselves. In addition, medical compliance is complicated by medical culture's production of physicians who may feel epistemically superior to their patients (more on this in Chapter 6), an attitude that may be picked up by patients and can impede a patient-centered approach to care: a recent study shows that a significant number of patients are afraid to question their physicians, not wanting to be viewed as "difficult" (Frosch et al. 2012). This concern, plus patients' perception that their physicians are being authoritarian, produces compliance where perhaps it not ought to be (as I go on to argue).

Because the concepts of compliance and noncompliance are so negatively weighted in value and meaning, it has been proposed that we think instead of patient "adherence." Jeffrey Aronson, for instance, notes that the term "concordance" has been proposed as a substitute for "compliance" (Aronson 2007). He rejects that term as well, though, because its meaning is too similar to compliance. Aronson prefers "adherence," and, indeed, medical students in North America generally are taught that this is the proper term for current medical practices. Adherence refers to the persistence of patients to stick to a regime of medication as prescribed by their physicians. This change, some believe, might eventually weaken the paternalistic quality in physicians' efforts to gain patient compliance. The term "adherence" is thought to better emphasize relationship, collaboration, and respect. Paula Vuckovich distinguishes between the two terms, arguing that they function at two different levels: compliance is politically incorrect but sometimes is the sole aim, as with mental patients, whereas adherence is preferable and involves the patient's active participation in her own treatment program (Vuckovich 2010, 78). But in fact, the World Health Organization defines adherence as "The extent to which a person's behavior, taking medication, following a diet, and/ or executing lifestyle changes, corresponds with agreed recommendations from a health care provider" (Ngoh 2009, 132). As Vuckovich notes, in theory, "adherence" is sought, but in practice, compliance is the aim (2010, 78).

The desire for compliance in health care is not merely an exercise of authority between practitioners and their patients. Compliance is a concern of the health care industry because noncompliance takes a significant toll on patients' health and on a nation's economy. For example, regarding all diagnoses (not just psychiatric): "Research suggests that only about 50% of patients typically take their medications as prescribed, and only 50 to 60% of patients are adherent to prescribed medications over a 1-year period" (Ngoh 2009, 134). Indeed, Kleinsinger states that noncompliant behavior is probably one of the most common causes of treatment failure (Kleinsinger 2010, 54) and, as discussed in Section 1.5, the patient has been thought to be the source of the "problem of compliance" (WHO 2003). But before I discuss noncompliance, I will bring in a seemingly clear-cut and simple juxtaposition to compliance: the right to refuse treatment.

1.2 The right to refuse treatment

The Patient Self Determination Act was passed by U.S. Congress in 1990. This law gives patients the right to refuse treatment, among other things. Whereas the compliant patient agrees to a treatment plan and follows through on it, and the noncompliant patient assents to, or gives the impression of assenting to, the clinician's recommendations and then, for various reasons, does not follow through, the patient who is exercising his or her right to refuse treatment does so from the outset of the recommendations. Patients refuse treatment for all sorts of reasons, such as not considering their situation dire enough or preferring not to experience the side effects of a recommended medication.

Patient values play a central role in patients' decisions to refuse treatment. So do patients' feelings of ambivalence about diagnosis or treatment (Centorrino et al. 2001, 380). Ambivalence can give rise to unwillingness to follow doctors' orders. For example, patients diagnosed with Borderline Personality Disorder may not easily accept their diagnosis and so reject the clinician's efforts to change behaviors such as self-harming ones. Patients recently diagnosed with an early stage of paranoid schizophrenia may, on the one hand, suspect something is wrong with them and, on the other hand, be suspicious of the psychiatrists who are doing the diagnosing. Or, a patient who believes the FBI inserted a chip into her brain in order to control her thoughts may both fear taking medications because she is being told not to trust the doctor and desire relief from the relentless control she experiences. Some bipolar patients go off their medications because they miss the zest and creative edge they experience when not taking medication. However, it is an open question whether or not such patients should be viewed as noncompliant or simply as exercising their right to refuse treatment. As Deborah Spitz points out, psychiatrists do not usually talk in terms of "refusal" unless that refusal places the patient at immediate risk if she is not treated. For example, a pregnant woman who is depressed and refuses anti-depressants is usually met with respect for her decision, but if a pregnant woman who is suicidal and psychotic refuses medication and is deemed to be at immediate risk, the court usually is asked to intervene.[1] Yet state laws vary with regard to what constitutes legal justification for intervention. For example, although not a psychiatric case, one of the most renowned recent cases comes from Texas, where 33-year-old pregnant Marlise Munoz became brain dead after a blood clot formed in her lung. Her husband and parents were prepared to honor Munoz's wish not to be technologically sustained if she were brain dead. However, Texas law required that, because she was pregnant, Munoz's wishes were irrelevant, and the life of the fetus required that the body of Munoz be sustained (Fernandez and Eckholm 2014; the HUB 2014).

When it comes to forced treatment for psychiatric patients, the question of patients' rights becomes very complex. Elyn Saks says that mental health clinicians tend to view psychotropic drugs as the salvation for patients and patient refusals of medication as a product of their illness, whereas lawyers tend to view refusals in terms of patient autonomy as an exercise of their refusal (Saks 2002, 84). She asks "Why does the state get to choose medication—with all that that entails—rather than suffering and disability" (Saks 2002, 86). Although Saks supports forced medications under the limiting condition of patient incompetence, she says that "the typical reasons patients refuse medication generally do not reflect incompetence and are worthy of respect" (Saks 2002, 96). In addition, giving patients a robust right to refuse medications can be beneficial to the therapeutic relationship (Saks 2002, 88). Saks points out that, for various reasons, some patients may prefer to be ill, and so "we should not forcibly medicate people for the sake of restoring them to mental health solely because they are impaired, not themselves, and likely to benefit from treatment" (Saks 2002, 89). The right to refuse treatment is not straightforward, as this discussion is beginning to show. In general, though, when a patient is refusing treatment, in addition to evaluating that patient's competence, it is important for psychiatrists to consider whether the treatment explanation is complete, whether the patient really understands, whether the patient feels asked, and whether the patient is disagreeing but not saying so explicitly.[2] Then, unless the patient is incompetent, it is important to respect patients' decisions to stay mentally ill if they refuse treatment. By "respect" I do not mean that the psychiatrist should abandon attempts to help stabilize the patient, but, instead, to ease up on pressured persuasion while remaining in a trustful conversation. (See Halpern [2001] for a discussion on the shortcomings of respecting patient autonomy.) I call attention to these issues because patients who have refused treatment and are forced to receive it, or who feel coerced into acquiescing to medications, may act defiantly. Clinicians need to be cautious, in responding to defiance, that they appropriately respect patients' behavior when that defiance is itself an appropriate response. What, exactly, this claim entails (I will call it "giving uptake") is the sort of messy question I will unpack in the following chapters.

1.3 Noncompliance

As it is typically understood in medicine, noncompliance occurs when a patient agrees to a treatment plan but does not follow through on it. According to research, noncompliance occurs when the patient is in denial, is depressed, is drug-dependent, is demented, or when cultural differences or cost of treatment become an issue (Kleinsinger 2010, 56). As we have seen, however, patients may be noncompliant when they agree to take medications only because they feel coerced into taking them. Thus, the right to refuse treatment and noncompliance are complicated when clinicians are coercive, or when patients experience them as coercive, or when patients are not competent to share in decision-making.

One way in which the right to refuse treatment and noncompliant behavior are intertwined is with respect to children. First of all, as Robert Kruger explains, the line between noncompliance and right of refusal is blurred because children generally are not thought of as having the legal right to consent or not consent.[3] The legal responsibility for decision-making for children falls to the parents or guardians. Parents often find it extremely difficult—and sometimes impossible—to force a child to go to therapy or take their medications, if the child refuses. Kruger's experiences in child psychiatry lead him to say that the interesting questions regarding the blurred boundaries between the concepts of refusal and noncompliance concern the reasons the child refuses. Some children refuse medications because they are worried that they will change the child's self-conception; others refuse because they dislike swallowing pills; others believe the problem is not with them but with their parents. Some children are compliant when talking with the psychiatrist but refuse treatment when they get home. And some children do not want to go to therapy because they do not think there is anything wrong with them. Others do not want to go to therapy because they are worried about the potential for being stigmatized if their peers find out. The paradox is that caregivers who are the legally consenting agents may be compliant on behalf of their noncompliant, or refusing, child. Thus, the relevance of thinking about these concepts in terms of Wittgenstein's family resemblances is highlighted when we consider them in relation to child psychiatry. From the perspective of medicine, it is noncompliance that requires explanation, and, regarding adults as well as children, the *reasons* for noncompliance are often the interesting part, as Kruger notes.

Although noncompliance is typically thought of as a way to frame a patient's failure to follow through on a treatment plan, I call attention to the fact that noncompliance sometimes is an attitude a patient takes that may or may not result in noncompliant actions. This point is important with respect to defiant people as well. A patient may be noncompliant, or defiant, toward psychiatrists (or, indeed, any person in an authoritative position, as I will argue in Chapter 2) as a way to defend against being overpowered or manipulated by the combined forces of the institution of medicine and their socialization. Noncompliant or defiant attitudes, Marilyn Frye suggests, may help patients make more critically informed decisions, including whether or not to comply with psychiatrists' treatment protocol. That is, a noncompliant or defiant attitude may or may not lead to noncompliant or defiant actions.[4] As I argue in this book, defiance may also be grounded in poverty, racism, sexism, transphobia, and other sources of social stratification that impede, and often prevent, the possibility of living a flourishing life. It also may arise from living lives filled with despair, suffering, or distraction (such as mothers without help or support might face).

This distinction is important because it can lead to different results. Therefore, this is a good moment for me to clarify the language—and also the underlying concepts—I will be using with regard to noncompliant and defiant attitudes and actions. I will sometimes separate defiant attitudes from defiant actions, while at other times I will use the term "defiant behavior." I do this because I think that, most of the time, defiance includes both attitudes and actions (the good, the bad, and the kind that is caused by mental illness). Nevertheless, the assumption found in most medical literature is that when the health care team talks about a patient's noncompliance, they are referring to the patient's action (or inaction, to be precise).

In terms of explanations as to why psychiatric patients are noncompliant, I focus on four themes: lack of health literacy (Ngoh 2009); inability to refill prescriptions or lack of desire to refill them (Olfson et al. 2000; personal observations at Emergency Psychiatric Services); psychoanalytic resistance theory; and reactance theory (Fogarty and Youngs 2000). See Box 1.1 for reasons why psychiatric patients discontinue their medications. Let me remind readers that the aim here is to show how these concepts are at play in psychiatry both separately and together, thereby paving the way for a discussion of defiance as distinct from all of these forms of noncompliance, yet not wholly distinct.

Box 1.1 Reasons why psychiatric patients discontinue their medications

- Drug-related adverse effects
- Short-term relief from depression, or, conversely, the lack of relief
- Reluctance to take pills
- Depression itself as a factor for nonadherence to medical treatment
- Lack of physician/patient communication
- Social stigma
- Poor commitment to treatment
- Lack of patient education
- Spousal separation, death of a spouse, or divorce
- Lack of social support
- Complexity and behavioral demands of concurrent restrictions such as weight loss or smoking cessation
- Exacerbation of a comorbid condition (Ruoff 2005)

1.4 **Explanations for noncompliance in psychiatric patients**

1.4.1 **Health literacy**

Health literacy is defined as "the degree to which individuals have the capacity to obtain, process, and understand basic health information and services needed to make appropriate health decisions. Thus, health literacy relates to both the cognitive and functional skills used to make health-related decisions" (Ngoh 2009, 134). Patients who have poor health literacy are less likely to follow doctors' orders, as I will illustrate through a discussion of the case of the Lee family in Section 1.6.2. I call attention to the point here that the interpretation of a patient's lack of health literacy gets messy when clinicians are evaluating patients whose cultural norms make it seem as if they lack health literacy when, in fact, they may be exercising their right to refuse treatment.

On the other hand, patients who do not perform the "good patient role" are not always noncompliant deliberately or with good reason. Sometimes, for example, their current state impedes their reasoning. Patients who have delusions may decide not to take the medications prescribed by their psychiatrist because they do not believe there is something wrong with their belief system. For the purposes of the discussion at this point, I use definitions by the American Psychiatric Association (2013; 1994) and Kaliuzhna et al, who define delusions as "beliefs that are rationally untenable beliefs based on incorrect inference about reality. These beliefs persist despite the evidence to the contrary and are not ordinarily accepted by other members of the person's culture or subculture" (Kaliuzhna et al. 2012, e34771).

People can be deluded about body image, for example. Distortions of body image are found in patients with anorexia nervosa, whose subjective experience of their body is as fat, but whose height and weight show that they are, in fact, underweight (according to objective calculations of Body Mass Index [BMI]). According to Espeset et al. (2012), delusional thinking about body image is present when the patient cannot recognize that she is severely underweight and, instead, clings to the notion that her subjective experience is correct. One patient, Frida, whose BMI is 14, says:

> I've had big problems accepting that I've been diagnosed with anorexia. Cause people with anorexia are very thin, and I'm not. So then it doesn't fit me. And when I look at myself in the mirror I really can't understand where I have anorexia. It's nowhere! (Espeset et al. 2011, 185)

Frida and others with this form of distorted body image say they may start to feel "crazy" when others point out the gap between subjective and objective reality, but still hold firm to their own beliefs about their body. Anorexic patients who are delusional about their body weight are frequently noncompliant about prescribed structured eating and injunctions not to over-exercise. While current evidence indicates that people with delusions can, with cognitive behavioral therapy, change their beliefs (and thus, defining delusions as "fixed beliefs" is incorrect), it is nevertheless the case that many deluded patients hold entrenched beliefs that are resistant to change (Kaliuzhna et al. 2012). This can lead to noncompliance. While health literacy can, in many cases, be improved through therapy and education, it may be limited by the degree of the patient's impairment.

1.4.2 Problems refilling prescriptions

Other patients are noncompliant with doctors' orders to take their medications, but the reason is that they are unable to refill their prescriptions. For some patients, their noncompliance may not include a noncompliant attitude; in fact, they may want to follow the treatment plan but, due to problems in living, are unable to do so. Problems range from not having transportation to a location where they can refill their prescriptions, to not having insurance or their own money to pay for them, to impairment in judgment such that they are unable to calculate the costs and benefits of continuing their medications once the initial prescription is gone. Again, whether or not these problems constitute noncompliance depends on how we define it and how the definition relates to such patients.

For example, one way that quality of care is evaluated is by outcome-based measures. "Compliance with prescribed medications is an intermediate outcome measure that assumes a positive health outcome will follow for the patient who follows the regime" (Morris and Schultz 1993, 593). However, as Morris and Schultz say, questions of compliance and noncompliance may be beside the point, from the patient's perspective. Patients appear to take or refuse to take their medicine based on non-pharmacological values, such as economic, psychological, interpersonal, and social ones. Such processes in decision-making about whether or not to take prescribed medications seem to make the concepts of compliance and noncompliance irrelevant to the patient. The cost of medications, for example, may put out of reach the patient's ability to fill a prescription, placing out of the patient's control any question of compliance. The need for self-regulation and agency may lead patients to alter the regime, such as taking more or less than prescribed in order to experience a sense of control. Some patients consider a prescription as an indication of the quality of the interpersonal relationship between the patient and the physician: sometimes as a gesture of concern, which interpretation leads to compliance; and sometimes as a dismissal—medication as a replacement for genuine engagement with the patient's travails—which interpretation leads to noncompliance. Even when patients were looking for a therapeutic outcome, the one they aimed at often was not the measure set by theory. For instance, if the patient's goal in taking a medication was to be able to return to work, and she was unable to do so, then she counted the medication as having failed in therapeutic value even if she received some relief from pain and discomfort from the medication. These patient values especially are important to consider when we are querying why psychiatric patients do not take their medications properly, if at all.

The conflict between clinicians and patients with respect to medication compliance is unlikely to go away until patients' values are taken into account. As Morris and Schultz put it:

> Trostle [another researcher] has proposed that, "Noncompliance is an unavoidable byproduct of collisions between the clinical world and other competing worlds of work, play, friendship, and family life." People who take medicine live in these worlds continuously; they are patients intermittently. Outcomes research on medicine taking will have value only to the degree that it recognizes and accepts these worlds as vital components of the patient's perspective. (Morris and Schultz 1993, 605)

These collisions may seem like plain noncompliance to the psychiatrist, but may in some cases be the exercise of good defiance. That is, sometimes a patient has to be defiant in order to uphold his values. As I will explain in the following chapters, defiance is not the same as noncompliance, but is related to it.

1.4.3 Psychoanalytic resistance

Defiance is often misunderstood as unconscious dysfunctional psychic resistance. But the concept of resistance is also misunderstood. "Resistance" is a psychoanalytic term introduced by Freud. In order to distinguish between psychoanalytic theories of resistance and what I am calling "good" defiance, I need briefly to examine the evolution of the concept of resistance from Freudian thought through current ideas. Roughly, Freud's interpretation of behavior (such as noncompliance or undermining of the therapeutic alliance) is that a part of the patient is being "defiant" because he or she "does not want to get better." For early Freudians, such behavior constituted unconscious resistance to healing, a "digging in of one's heels" in the throes of illness—a fist holding on to what is familiar. As Mitchell and Black explain, Freud's hypothesis was that certain memories and feelings are too disturbing and incompatible with the rest of consciousness and so are repressed (Mitchell and Black 1995, 4). In the therapeutic relationship, those resistances show up in transferences to the psychoanalyst. Freud believed that the work of healing precisely was to focus on the patient's resistance because it was the source of neurosis.

There has been a theoretical shift from Freud to self-psychology (cf. Gammelgaard 2003 for a review). Freud's theory of resistance and transference did not require a conception of the self; instead, he theorized these defenses in terms of ego states. Ego analysts, following the work of Heinz Hartmann (1964), aimed to resolve ambiguities in Freud's theory of the ego by introducing the concept of the self, a concept that helped unify the ego states and enabled better understanding of non-neurotic patients. Self-psychologists, among many other contributions, proposed an *adaptive* interpretation of patients who manifest internal struggles: the idea is that equilibrium disturbance does not feel good and, as a result, keeping something out of awareness is adaptive. Allan Schore explains that the "developing infant's regulatory transactions with the selfobject allows for the maintenance of its internal homeostatic equilibrium" (Schore 2002, 436). Sometimes, something is too overwhelming to see; therefore, we adapt by keeping that thing out of awareness. Heinz Kohut's (1971) work is seminal in this theoretical shift away from dysfunctional resistance and toward adaptive internal balance. Kohut emphasizes the psyche's efforts to maintain or re-establish equilibrium. For example, he discusses the creative act as an internal need to express feelings that "propel the individual toward a solution" that gives pleasure, "which is the emotional accompaniment of the suddenly restored narcissistic balance" (Kohut 1971, 316). Self-regulation is the work of the internal self-structures, and balance is the aim.

As Schore says, self-psychology represents a substantial shift from a Freudian focus on the ego and the "intrapsychic unconscious to a relational unconscious whereby the unconscious mind of one communicates with the unconscious mind of another" (2009, 190). Schore's aim is to integrate the disciplines of psychoanalysis and neuroscience, and he offers a nonconscious understanding of early development of psychopathology that is interdisciplinary. It is instructive to look at self-psychology in order to better understand what in later chapters I describe as "good defiance." For some people, defiance is a way they respond and adapt; therefore, self-regulation gets expressed in various ways depending on the individual. Adaptive defiance is good in that it is adaptive, but it is not the kind I am most interested in. The difference between the sort of defiance I advocate, and self-psychology's relational unconscious and the need of the self to maintain or re-establish balance and equilibrium, is a matter of theorizing defiance as constitutively grounded in external relationality coupled with its conscious knowing and telling. Much more needs to be said in order to clarify the difference between the two (my theory of defiance and that of adaptive establishment of self-equilibrium), but my theorizing is postponed until later chapters.

1.4.4 **Reactance theory**

A fourth theme in the literature on noncompliance in psychiatric patients can be found in the psychological theory of "reactance." This theory developed to explain why people sometimes do the opposite of what they are asked to do (harking back to the passage by Dostoevsky in Section 1.1). It differs from psychoanalytic resistance theory in that it assumes the patient to be intentional and deliberate in her reactance. The idea is that we believe we have some degree of freedom in choices and actions, and that we value those freedoms enough to try to protect them. Brehm and Brehm (2013) suggested that a threat to our freedoms would motivate us to try to re-establish the jeopardized freedom. How reactant a person is depends on "the value the individual placed on the freedom, the number of freedoms imperiled, and the perceived severity of the menace" (Fogarty and Youngs 2000, 2367).

In medicine, reactance theory is applied to the finding that many people believe that the change in lifestyle advocated by their doctors is going to impinge on important freedoms. Here, again, the role of coercion may play a part. Fogarty and Youngs found that physician–patient interactions influence patient reactance in two ways: (a) the tone of voice that the physician uses in giving advice, and (b) the perception of the patient that he or she has the ability to choose (a sense of freedom) with respect to treatment options. Threats trigger reactance and, in turn, noncompliance (Fogarty and Youngs 2000, 2369). Reactance may occur even when the patient's perception of coercion is mistaken, as when the patient has internalized the good patient role and so, on the one hand, wishes to be compliant, but, on the other hand, feels trapped by her own inclination to be compliant and so sees the physician as coercive. But others, such as some psychiatric patients, actually do have important freedoms taken away, as when doctors involuntarily hospitalize them, use restraints on them, or put them in locked seclusion. In such cases, patients may argue that they are justifiably noncompliant. Once again, we see that clear and distinct boundaries cannot be maintained between the various concepts under discussion—including hard distinctions between reactance theory and the self-psychology movement that emerged out of a theory of psychoanalytic resistance.

1.5 **Reframing noncompliance**

As I have shown, many reasons exist for patient noncompliance. Noncompliant patients typically are viewed through a lens of frustration, negative judgment, disapproval, and, sometimes, blame when their own illnesses are causing themselves—and others—distress. What is especially interesting to me, though, are the times when patients consciously and deliberately refuse to be good, cooperative, or (normatively) appropriately self-interested. It will become clear that both the assessment of, and accountability for, deliberate noncompliance is a central problem to delve into in chapters to come.

The problem with reactance theory and other explanations for noncompliance is that many of them still frame noncompliance as the patient's "fault," in that an explanation for the failure to "comply" is sought in the patient's world, singling him or her out as the "cause" of being difficult. What I mean by this is that many theories of noncompliance fail to contextualize the problem, and so neglect the role that institutions and systems play in producing the need for noncompliance. For example, reactance theory, although recognizing the patient's perspective, does not capture the context of the patient in relation to the broader institution of psychiatry. In contrast, I will introduce the concept of defiance as a virtue. In doing so, I take some expressions of reasonable and deliberate noncompliance to be a good form of defiance. Note that here I have slipped in two central modifiers: "reasonable" and "deliberate." What constitutes each of these characteristics will be developed in following chapters. Note also that, while I defer defining the concept of defiance until Chapter 2, noncompliance and defiance, although logically separable, often seem to slide together in attitude and action.

Setting noncompliance within a larger societal framework also highlights the importance of trust, which Misztal says is "an active political accomplishment" (Misztal 1996, 7, quoted in Tauber 2007, 42). Tauber (2007) argues that the failure in medicine to be considered a trusted institution is a sign of a social crisis where our "communal glue" is coming undone. "The patient's best interests" are not being protected, and mistrust may be the result. Mistrust especially is the case in the field of psychiatry where, despite the overwhelming numbers of good and dedicated clinicians, public perceptions of psychiatry continue to suffer from worries that it is a form of social control, that it is not a genuine science, and that psychiatrists are tampering with the freedoms of the different and deviant in society.

This is especially going to be the case if people deviate from social norms for expected behavior, beliefs, and attitudes and thus are treated as if they are irrational or a danger to self or others. Mistrust of psychiatrists and the field of psychiatry is part of a broader phenomenon in society of downtrodden or disadvantaged people's mistrust of authority. This mistrust is not only a matter of various laws and patient rights, or of fear and resentment toward misuses of authority, but also of the norms that underlie them (see Box 1.2 for an explanation of norms). As I argue in later chapters, norms for how to behave, including how to be a good patient, are produced and structured by dominant culture; they permeate our understanding not only of how we ought to think and act but also how we experience and interpret others. An analysis of norms and how they constrict movement is a theme in this book, and an understanding of the link between dominant norms and defiance will aid clinicians in responding appropriately to expressions of defiance.

Box 1.2 What are norms, where do they come from, and what justifies them?

Brennan et al. (2013) distinguish between formal and informal norms. Formal norms are ones such as legal norms, which typically vary from state to state and nation to nation. Formal norms are enforced by an authoritative body that has the power to interpret and enforce these norms and provides a rational reason for people to comply—namely, fear of punishment (Brennan et al. 2013, 5). Informal norms typically lack such explicitness and are not legally enforceable, but people who violate them can be shunned, ridiculed, or unforgiven. They discuss only informal social and moral norms, but I also include linguistic, epistemic, and practical reasoning norms. Brennan et al. argue that norms are not merely social practices such as conventions and customs, nor are they merely clusters of desires: norms are clusters of normative *attitudes plus knowledge of those attitudes*. They explicate this definition as having two requirements: that a significant number of a group (not all) holds normative attitudes about some norm (the Attitude Condition); and that a significant number of a group (not all) knows that a significant number of a group holds those normative attitudes about that norm (the Knowledge Condition). The groups of people who meet either the Attitude or the Knowledge Condition of a given norm might not overlap; the point is that norms are, to a significant degree, group norms. Readers might object to the Knowledge Condition on the grounds that many, if not most, norms in everyday life seem to be followed unconsciously or at least not deliberatively. Brennan et al. explain that the reason the Knowledge Condition is important is that it would be odd to claim that a norm exists (and therefore ought to be followed)

(continued)

and yet for no one to know about it. This understanding of norms also does not require that all people within a particular group endorse a given norm, a point that this book highlights with respect to defiance (Brennan et al. 2013, 29–34). Brennan et al. say that the purpose of a norm is to hold people accountable to one another (Brennan et al. 2013, 36). In sum, then, these two conditions highlight the beliefs, judgments, expectations, and attitudes that a group deploys or attributes, and that signify "what matters to us, who we take ourselves to be, and how we see ourselves and others," thereby expressing what we hold one another accountable for (Brennan et al. 2013, 37).[5]

1.6 **Two problem cases**

In this section, I present two problem sorts of cases in order to illustrate the challenge that psychiatrists and other clinicians face when trying to interpret people's behavior and sort out appropriate responses. These cases are fodder for thought and are not meant to provide definitive direction. The first type of case raises a problem in treatment of patients with anorexia nervosa (AN), namely whether they have the right to refuse treatment when they present a danger to themselves (i.e., where treatment would involve forced feeding to save their lives), and whether to consider a refusal to follow doctors' orders to take in a certain number of calories as acts of noncompliance. This psychiatric and health problem illustrates the blurred edges of noncompliance, the right to refuse treatment, and the right to choose death under certain circumstances. Then, in Section 1.6.2, I sketch out a narrative familiar to many readers, Anne Fadiman's *The Spirit Catches You and You Fall Down* (1997). This case illustrates the convergence of care-seeking, noncompliance, cultural clashes, and paternalism.

1.6.1 **Anorexia nervosa and the right to refuse treatment**

The demand for women to meet the norms of feminine beauty gives rise to some frightening practices both on the medical front and in women's lives (Hesse-Biber 2006). Kathryn Morgan shows how Western medical technologies employ disciplinary practices to enforce a standard of thinness that campaigns against obesity (Morgan 2011). Fat hatred and the campaign against obesity drives many women to desperate measures, including refusing to eat and having bariatric surgery on their stomachs to decrease eating. As Morgan says, "weight loss surgeons operate on completely healthy stomachs situated in the bodies of pathologized individuals, technically creating a dangerously dysfunctional digestive track while describing the fat surgical subject as "morbid" and "monstrous"" (Morgan 2011, 207). Some women take this route to thinness while others engage in starvation.

Anorexia nervosa (AN) is a mental disorder with a high mortality rate (Papadopoulos et al. 2009). It is the third most common chronic disorder among North American adolescent girls, after obesity and asthma (Robb et al. 2002, 1347; American Psychiatric Association 2000). A longitudinal study by Folios et al. found that people with AN in their research cohort had a sixfold increased mortality compared with the general population (Papadopoulos et al. 2009, 14). Although suicide was the greatest cause of death among people with anorexia, the disorder itself was the next highest cause (Papadopoulos et al. 2009). In another study, researchers found that the highest mortality in patients with AN was found with patients whose BMI fell below 11.5 (Rosling et al. 2011, 309). It is hypothesized that people (mostly women; DSM V, 341) become anorexic for a number of reasons. Primary among them are an intense and overwhelming fear of becoming fat and feeling fat as a result of distorted body image. Yet even this explanation is incomplete; for example, Morag Macsween argues that women with AN are attempting to transform the degraded feminine body by disciplining their desires, giving a sociopolitical perspective on AN in women (Macsween 1993). Additionally, it has been hypothesized that AN is more likely to be found in fat-phobic societies such as the U.S. and some European countries, but that idea is not supported by evidence (Watters 2010, ch. 1; Lee 2001; Rieger et al. 2001; Simpson 2002). Force-feeding is a common treatment therapy for patients with AN who are experiencing organ failure and other life-threatening health problems.

Compulsory feeding usually happens in a hospital. Therefore, I take a brief step back to discuss service users' experiences of involuntary hospitalization, and then I relate some of their points to involuntary feeding. One of the most frightening experiences for psychiatric patients is involuntary commitment—and, I will add, involuntary treatments such as forced feeding. As John Mack explains, the feeling that we have some personal power to create and govern our own lives is essential to our sense of self: "One of the most disturbing aspects of being hospitalized for medical or psychiatric reasons is the loss of the sense of agency, power, and autonomy" (Mack 1997, 563). This sense of loss and fear is amplified when hospitalization is against one's will. To compound these problems, service users know that they may experience being sexually molested and physically and mentally abused, and that reporting on abuses may be ignored (Garrett and Posey 1997, 203). The authors add that service users' fears of commitment are real and serious, and that "unless we are willing to own up to that fact, consumer [service user] opposition to commitment laws will continue" (Garrett and Posey 1997, 206).

I apply these comments from Garrett and Posey to people with AN who—perhaps voluntarily and perhaps involuntarily—are hospitalized for treatment. It is not hard to imagine the helplessness, sense of violation, and powerlessness experienced by someone who refuses to eat and yet is subjected to feeding against her will. Even under threat of death, some people with AN would reject being force-fed, to the degree that they attempt to pull out the technologies that supply nutrition. How are we to interpret such behavior? I suggest that this legal and ethical problem exemplifies the difficulty in sorting out the different ways of understanding patients' behavior such as noncompliance, exercising the right to refuse treatment, or being defiant. Furthermore, if patients with AN refuse nutritional treatment and rip out wires and tubes that provide nutrition, they could be exhibiting good defiance, bad defiance, or neither—because they are mentally ill (I develop these distinctions in Chapter 2).

Heather Draper (2000) argues that, under certain circumstances, people with anorexia should be permitted to refuse forced feeding even if it results in death. Draper says that, in some cases, forced feeding indicates a failure to respect a competent refusal of therapy, arguing that the right to refuse treatments, even if the likely result is death, is one that we recognize in many other types of cases (Draper 2000). Draper is sensitive to the difficulty of making a claim for a right to refuse treatment when it applies to patients with AN, but she points out that one controversy involves the conception of AN as a mental disorder, where a refusal to eat to the point of endangering one's life is by definition irrational. Draper challenges this equation. She says that "It is undoubtedly awful to watch someone—possibly a young someone—die when they can so easily be saved. However, if justice is to be given to those sufferers who can neither live with their anorexia nor live without it, we must listen carefully to their refusals of therapy" (Draper 2000, 133). Draper argues that the patient's assessment of her or his quality of life should be the determining factor in whether or not to force-feed someone.

Because many AN individuals feel coerced and compromised by psychiatrists and other clinicians, they have established what are called "pro-ana" (pro-anorexia) websites. These websites serve as a sanctuary where an anorexic lifestyle can be supported safely while providing an underground resistance movement to psychiatric and social models of disease (Fox, Ward, and O'Rourke 2005). For example, one poster writes:

> What does pro-ED [pro-ana] mean to me? People with eating disorders are isolated
> and surrounded by people who don't understand what we think or feel.... Some of

us need our EDs still and aren't ready to recover. Eating disorders are dangerous, and ignorance compounds that. We can't go ask for safe advice from non-EDs without a risk of being hospitalized or shunned. Pro-ED to me means understanding that there's no shame in how we are, and acceptance that this is how we will continue to be for an indefinite period of time. It means support for us so we don't have to deal with this alone. It means nonjudgmental help so we can survive and remain as safe and healthy as possible while maintaining the behaviors we still need to keep. Pro-ED to me does not mean recruiting, encouraging or teaching others to be anorexic, encouraging excessively dangerous practices, or starving to death. (Anonymous, Dias 2003, 38)

I do not attempt to settle the ethical and social questions that arise from the discussion on AN in this book. Instead, I merely want to show how complex the various bioethical and normative issues are when we consider the voices of anorexic patients and how difficult it is to separate out the distinction between the right to refuse treatment and one of the physician's core responsibilities: to save lives. The question that lurks is not only one of when to intervene with respect to patients with psychiatric illnesses, but also of how to conceptualize the possibilities of competency and the expressions of potentially good defiance.

In Section 1.6.2, I present a narrative that is not specific to the psychiatric domain but that extends questions of family resemblances and blurred boundaries between concepts. This narrative, of the Hmong Lee family in California in the 1980s, illustrates how cultural clashes can make assessments of noncompliance and appropriate responses to cultural and ethnic differences challenging indeed.

1.6.2 Noncompliance, a culture clash, and assumptions within Western medicine: The story of the Lee family

Lia Lee was born in 1982 to a Hmong family that emigrated to Merced County in the United States. Hundreds of Hmong refugees had fled the Laotian regime in the late 1970s and early 1980s, and, at the time, one in five residents in Merced County was Hmong. Between the ages of eight months and four and a half years, Hmong child Lia Lee was admitted to hospital seventeen times and visited the emergency room or outpatient pediatrics more than 100 times (Fadiman 1997, 38). Lia had a very severe seizure disorder that required constant medical attention, and her parents recognized the urgency when she seized. Yet in Hmong culture, Anne Fadiman explains, the attitude toward such phenomena was not purely medical and alarmist. The Lees' understanding of Lia's situation followed Hmong beliefs that *qaug dab peg*—or "the spirit catches you and you fall down"—is a soul-stealing spirit that is considered both dangerous and blessed. Those afflicted by *qaug dab peg* are thought to be touched by the divine and often become shamans as adults, having a special capacity for healing and empathy. Lia's parents, therefore, treasured and pampered their child according to Hmong practices even while appealing to Western medicine to assist them with medical interventions.

Because Lia's seizures lasted so long and left her unconscious with the potential for brain damage, Lia was placed on a medical regimen that became increasingly complicated. It included several different drugs, in both pill and liquid form, of varying dosages to be given at different times of the day—a confusing treatment plan even to a medically sophisticated patient. The Lees were illiterate and spoke virtually no English. They could not read or follow the instructions on the labels. Public health nurses tried myriad ways to help the Lees administer the proper medicines, including creative visual charts and color-coded bottles, but the Lees could not or would not follow the treatment plan. Lia's condition grew worse.

Neil Ernst and Peggy Philp were the two supervising pediatricians who served in the front line of defense whenever Lia's parents brought her to the emergency room. They were dedicated and committed physicians who struggled with strong emotions as their efforts to provide the best medical attention possible seemed to be repeatedly thwarted by the Lees. When Lia was one year old, Neil reported to the Health Department that "the mother states that she will not give the Dilantin at home. In addition, she also states that she has increased the child's Phenobarbital to 60 mg, b.i.d." (Fadiman 1997, 56). Later, the father refused to give Lia her Tegretol. Then they stopped giving her Phenobarbital. Both Neil and Peggy felt frustrated, enraged, powerless, and afraid for Lia's life. Not only were the Lees jeopardizing Lia's mental capabilities and, perhaps, her life, but they were neither deferential to the physicians nor appreciative of the largely voluntary nature of their efforts due to low reimbursement rates. Eventually, Neil reported the Lees to Child Protective Services for child abuse.

> [B]ecause of poor parental compliance regarding the medication this case obviously would come under the realm of child abuse, specifically child neglect....Unless there could be some form of compliance with the medication regimen and control of the child's seizure disorder, this child is at risk for status epilepticus which could result in irreversible brain damage and also possibly death. It is my opinion that this child should be placed in foster home placement so that compliance with medication could be assured. (Fadiman 1997, 58–9)

Lia was removed from her parents' home.

Although she was returned to her home some time later, Lia eventually died of complications from sepsis. Yet Fadiman argues in *The Spirit Catches You and You Fall Down* (1997) that she neither died of sepsis nor of noncompliance, but of a failure effectively to communicate across cultures. This was only in small part due to the language barrier: the only translator available was a janitor who did not speak Hmong but only a related language. The larger issues were the way most practitioners of the Western medical establishment at the time, as well as the Lee family, stayed entrenched in their own cultural ontology, value system, and phenomenology. As Dan Murphy, a family practice resident considered the most knowledgeable and interested in Hmong culture at the time, puts it:

> Until I met Lia I thought if you had a problem you could always settle it if you just sat and talked long enough. But we could have talked to the Lees until we were blue in the face—we could have sent the Lees to *medical school* with the world's greatest translator—and they would still think their way was right and ours was wrong. (Fadiman 1997, 259; emphasis in original)

Yet the problem was not only the seeming incommensurability, but also the long-standing practice in Western medicine of expecting patients and their families to adopt a particular stance toward practitioners—that of deference and compliance based on trust in their authority.

As Fadiman points out:

> [O]f the forty or so American doctors, nurses, and Merced County agency employees I spoke with who had dealt with Lia and her family, several had a vague idea that "spirits" were somehow involved, but Jeanine Hilt [a social worker who worked closely with the Lees] was the only one who had actually asked the Lees what they thought was the cause of their daughter's illness. (Fadiman 1997, 22)

This absence of nonjudgmental questions was not only a mistake in terms of how to deal with cultural clashes in medicine, but also evidence of an underlying assumption about the rightness of Western medicine's ways. One way that assumption shows up is in thinking that if the patient and her family do not follow doctors' advice and orders, they are being noncompliant. What is at stake when someone is considered noncompliant? Is it always bad to be that way? Is it ever a bad idea to be compliant, or is it always praiseworthy? And to what extent does compliance within medicine map onto cultural understandings of compliance in general society? On what norms and values are judgments of compliance and noncompliance based, and are they well grounded?

The situation in North America and Europe has improved significantly in recent decades, due in no small part to the educational efforts in the health care fields to require cultural competence. Physicians, nurses, social workers, and other practitioners make concerted efforts to understand their patients and to practice from a patient-centered perspective. Problems continue to emerge as new immigrant groups that practitioners are not yet familiar with enter developed countries. For example, there is a growing population of Somali refugees in Minnesota as well as in many other states and their different belief systems regarding obstetrics or healing from trauma present new challenges for practitioners (cf. Kroll, Yusuf, and Fujiwara 2010; Swetz et al. 2011; Scuglik et al. 2007; Wissink et al. 2005). To be clear, I do not take a relativist perspective either on cases of AN or of cultural differences; this point will be expanded on in later chapters. Nevertheless, judgments of non-compliance still occur with respect to cultural differences as well as the mentally ill and general societal norms. So, the questions I raised in this section are neither new nor resolved, but they represent some of the issues I take up in this book. I began this chapter with the medical concepts of compliance and noncompliance because they are central ethical and legal concepts in their own right—and because I take them to be part of a family of concepts in which defiance is found, along with concepts such as freedom, voice, resistance, and civil disobedience. I discuss the social importance of compliant behavior more generally in Chapter 2 when I develop the concept of defiance.

When is it rational to rebel, resist, and otherwise flaunt the edicts of authority? When is one's freedom, or sense of self, or subjectivity, being thwarted? These questions are crucial for the field of psychiatry to take up, because to fail to understand fully the complexity of patient noncompliance or defiance is to potentially (a) impede treatment; (b) make mistaken diagnoses; (c) reinforce the public and patients' mistrust of psychiatry; (d) perpetuate unjust hierarchies of power where the downtrodden or subjugated stand in a subordinate relation to authority; and (e) thwart the possibilities for flourishing and the ethical basis of society. Chapter 2 develops these points as I provide a theory of defiance for psychiatric patients.

Chapter 2

Theorizing defiance

2.1 Introduction and caveats

This chapter presents my general theory of defiance as a virtue. The overarching question is in what situation it is a good idea to refuse to live by what Nien Cheng calls "civilized virtues." Cheng was a political prisoner during the Cultural Revolution. She was placed in solitary confinement for more than six years, during which time she determined that virtues such as tolerance, forgiveness, and even humor were luxuries she could not easily afford (Cheng 1987, 218). In Chapter 1, I indicated that concepts such as compliance and noncompliance are partly normative, but there I focused on medical norms. In this chapter, I connect those concepts with cultural and social norms more generally, always keeping in mind that the purpose of this inquiry is to establish what sorts of norms are warranted in psychiatry.

Norms serve a primary function of fostering social relations, smoothing out tensions, and containing violence (see Box 1.2 on norms). Norms operate hegemonically. "Hegemony" is a way of talking about power relations that emphasizes the process by which a dominant group maintains its power—for example, through education, media, economics, social roles, and other methods of structuring and establishing norms and material existence. As I am using the term, "hegemony" assumes that the maintenance of domination is a struggle, and, thus, that the position of dominance is not a foregone conclusion—and is compatible with—indeed, constitutive of, true democratic practices. The United States, for example, is a hegemonic society in the sense that the ruling class primarily consists of white, heterosexual, upper-class males who maintain power through their control over institutions such as education, marriage, and medicine, while simultaneously are jostled and challenged by the voices of other, less privileged groups such as women of all colors, racialized people, gay people, working-class people, and immigrants. Thus, any discussion of deviance from norms, such as is involved in defiance, needs to include the roles of authority, complicity, and struggle in maintaining norms.

I emphasize to readers that this book is not going to cover a history of defiance in culture or provide a general analysis and application of it. Instead,

I am offering an examination of defiance toward an end that it is practical and useful in psychiatry. Doing so will require me to make use of concepts from philosophy and anthropology, such as domination, subjugation, oppression, and voice, as well as ideas about mental health and rationality as they intersect with epistemic and social arrangements in culture. This focus may sit uncomfortably with some clinicians, so I urge readers to approach this analysis in terms of systems and practices rather than in terms of individuals' failures within those structures. As I argue in Potter (2002)—drawing on Aristotle's claims about the relationship of the individual to the polis—when the overall structure of a system is less than virtuous, the individuals within it can only be so good; that is, our virtue as individual people is constrained by defective or ethically flawed health care systems. We need to keep this less personalized approach in mind as we identify problems with power and authority in psychiatry. Then, in Chapter 6, I bring home to readers the more particular applications to be made.

Because psychiatry is committed to the diagnosis and treatment of the mentally ill, thus serving a vulnerable and sometimes needy population with the aim of improving their lives, concepts such as oppression and voice may not seem relevant to this field. I hope to convince readers, though, that many patient populations not only subjectively experience themselves as oppressed, but that many of them are also objectively downtrodden and subjugated by a system that reinforces their status as inferior, less than fully human, or less deserving of treatment as equals.

2.2 **Aristotle's virtue ethics**

I take a loosely Aristotelian approach wherein virtue concerns both feelings and actions that a person's character expresses over time. By character, Aristotle means the sort of person we are and the way we have a tendency to respond when in particular situations. Our character includes not only the choices we make, but also the broader context in which they are seen as choiceworthy, such as the situation and persons involved, the background conditions that gave rise to needing to choose one way instead of another and, just as importantly, our own moral and epistemic strengths and weaknesses. Regarding the last point, I am referring specifically to our disposition or readiness to act in certain ways when we get into a given situation, and those past attitudes, feelings, and behaviors that make it more likely that we will act similarly in future similar situations. For example, if I have a tendency to blow up when faced with contractors who fail to keep their word, then if I think that is an ethically, socially, or pragmatically undesirable way to be, I will need to take into consideration my dispositional traits and try to change them instead of repeating them. Aristotelian virtue is also said to require practical reasoning, making virtue not only a moral quality of character, but an intellectual one. On Aristotle's view, virtue involves *phronesis*, a kind of practical reasoning that leads to decision-making toward right ends—ends that ultimately express flourishing for a human being. Aristotle's idea of *phronesis* is stronger than I subscribe to, so I set out features of practical reasoning that better provide a realistic standard in Chapter 5—ones that make a space for reasonable defiance to fall within the scope of a virtue.

Virtues are an intermediate between extremes. What Aristotle means is that each virtue has a deficient way of being that correlates with that virtue as well as an excessive way of being that correlates with that virtue. For example, one virtue is what Aristotle calls "mildness." Its scope is how we respond to insult and injury. Anger, Aristotle says, is an appropriate way to respond to insults and injury, either to oneself or to one's friends and family. But we can have a tendency toward too much anger (such as blowing up at people for minor insults, getting angry at those who did not do the wrong, holding grudges, seeking revenge) or too little anger (such as forgiving too quickly, being longsuffering, or sweeping things under the rug). The virtuous person aims at hitting the intermediate condition, where one's anger is expressed in proportion to the injury or insult, toward the person or institution that is believed to have done the wrong, with an appropriate aim in expressing that anger, and so on. I return to this way of understanding virtue in Chapter 3.

The reasons we need to develop virtues are twofold. First, virtues are good in themselves. Friendship is a virtue that is good to have "even if [we] had all the other goods" (Aristotle 2000, 1155a5). Additionally, on Aristotle's account, virtues contribute to *eudaimonia*—and not just for you or me, but for the neighborhood, the community, and society. What counts as the mean is contextual in that it is relative to me and it varies depending on the persons involved, the particularities of the situation, the parties' relation to power and authority, and so on. But virtues are not simply subjective—in each situation, a right way to feel and act exists, and feeling and acting within that mean is partly constitutive of flourishing. Of course, how virtues are understood depends on the historical context and societal needs at the time. For example, courage in ancient Greece focused on how and when to face fear in battle; Americans today might need courage to be whistle-blowers or to leave an abusive relationship or, as in the example of Traveling Thunder, to put the Whiteman in his place (see Section 2.3.2).

The classical conception of virtues presents a hopeful picture of flourishing individuals within a flourishing society. That is, the virtues arguably exist to enhance individual and social life within a well-functioning society (Plato 1974, 443d–e; Aristotle 2000). But most current societies are not well-functioning in that, although they may be efficient, or absent of overt internal violence, they still may be stratified, hierarchical, and shot through with unjust inequities. In a word, they are oppressive. I follow Marilyn Frye's definition of oppression as an unjust system of networks and barriers that catch people in all directions, molding and shaping them according to the benefit of a more powerful class of people, and reducing their choices and their freedom (Frye 1983). For example, structures of racism in the United States unjustly burden people of color while benefitting white people through what Peggy McIntosh calls an "invisible knapsack" of privileges (McIntosh 1988). According to Iris Marion Young, oppression and domination are two disabling constraints placed on certain social groups, including, for example, women, Blacks, Hispanic Americans, Native Americans, Jews, lesbians, gay men, transgendered people, Middle Easterners, Asians, working-class people, the elderly, and the physically and mentally disabled. By "disabling constraints," Young means the systematic and group-associated injustices that take the form of exploitation, marginalization, powerlessness, cultural imperialism, and violence (Young 2011). These forms of oppression and domination are disabling because they reduce, immobilize, and shape members of affected social groups in ways that drastically hinder their ability to live well. People who are considered to be mentally disabled are likely to experience the disabling effects of oppression within societies while at the same time may struggle with the disabling effects of mental illness. This is one of the groups I focus on in this book. But what it means to be "mentally disabled" is itself a contested idea, an issue I take up in later chapters.

Oppressive societies also affect the distribution and expression of virtue. As Claudia Card has argued, what are virtues for one group may be vices for another (Card 1990; cf. also Tessman 2005; Potter 2001). Long-standing—and often unconscious—patterns of benefits and burdens give rise to the socialization of people into different sets of virtues according to group memberships. I am interested in how the unequal distribution of virtues is played out with respect to the interpretation of and responses to defiant behavior within psychiatry. By highlighting the value of defiance for the downtrodden, members of oppressed groups, and the disenfranchised (including those disenfranchised by psychiatric disorders), I do not mean that defiance is not also valuable for others. But for most of this book my primary focus is on psychiatric norms as they intersect with variously positioned people. I argue that defiance is sometimes a necessary character trait in order for members of oppressed groups or those who face unjust authoritative power to live with self-respect. I call the readiness to be defiant a virtue. At the same time, I take seriously the potentially dire repercussions to the oppressed and others when they act defiantly—including the consequence that they may be diagnosed with a mental disorder, coerced into taking psychotropic medications, or hospitalized against their will. The concern is that medical and cultural matrices can collide when people seem to be defiant and that healthy virtuous defiance is sometimes conflated with bad, or even mad, behavior. So, it is important to get clear on how we think about, evaluate, and respond to behavior that we or others interpret as "defiant."

In Section 2.3, I first of all provide a conceptual analysis of defiance, setting it out as an attitude and behavior that responds to authoritative norms and structures as well as to authority figures. I distinguish it from civil disobedience, although I note that the two action-concepts share some features—in other words, they bear family resemblances. In Section 2.4, I argue that, under certain circumstances, defiance is a virtue. I draw on Lisa Tessman's theory of burdened virtues as a sustained thread throughout this book as I situate defiance as a virtue.

2.3 **The scope and content of defiance**

2.3.1 **Civility**

Political prisoner Cheng says in her memoir that there was no room for "civilizing virtues" while imprisoned during the Cultural Revolution. So I start the development of defiance as a virtue with a discussion of civility. Civility has a variety of understandings. Joan McGregor says it concerns good manners and "treating others as if they matter. The standards are those that go beyond the moral minimum; that is, they include more than merely not violating people's rights" (McGregor 2004, 26). Another kind of civility might be found in Cheshire Calhoun's idea of common decency. She argues that a minimally well-formed person will follow moral expectations that are neither obligatory nor supererogatory but that nevertheless a decent person would do. An example of decency is that of bringing a gift such as flowers, wine, or chocolates to the home of a host. To neglect such acts is not blameworthy, but it is not decent (Calhoun 2004). Jonathan Schonsheck argues that repudiating the central social values of tolerance and mutual respect is the most serious kind of incivility (Schonsheck 2004, 169). His idea is that "incivility escalates to insurrection, to civil war" (Schonsheck 2004, 175).

Civil behavior centered on values such as respect, tolerance, and decency may be hard to come by in societies with multiple oppressions; both those who misuse their structural power and those who receive such misuse or abuse may become defiant. I am making two points here. First, civility is a socializing mechanism that keeps people from revolting and people's tempers from undermining social relations; and second, what counts as civility varies depending on the group(s) with which one identifies or holds membership(s). Practically speaking, civility is a valuable social lubricant both with our peers and with those across class and culture divides. Still, civility is taken to be a virtue best exemplified and passed on by women (cf. Popenoe 2000; Noddings 1991), and those who fail to exhibit manners such as deference to authority are judged as morally flawed or mentally ill.

Defiance can be understood as a response to authority and, in particular, the way that authoritative bodies use power. Authoritative institutions and persons seem to call for deferential obedience but may overstep their bounds, especially if they use coercion to enforce their power. As Meir Dan-Cohen writes, "those subject to an authority are expected to defer to its wishes and demands. "Deference" signifies a "submission or yielding to the judgment, opinion, will, etc., of another," as well as an attitude of "respectful or courteous regard"" (Dan-Cohen 1994, 35). Authority, argues Dan-Cohen, seeks voluntary obedience by appealing to an attitude of respect for authority's claims on us (Dan-Cohen 1994, 35); being motivated by respect or regard expresses our willingness to accede to it. In other words, deference given by the ruled toward authority is a communicative act; it conveys the attitude that authoritative bodies expect the ruled to adopt. If those authoritative bodies use coercion to effect compliance, the attitude and motivation for being (freely) compliant is compromised (Dan-Cohen 1994, 38–9). Authorities' use of coercion may undercut its own legitimacy and may call for a challenge. One way to challenge coercive authority or abuse of authority is through defiance.

I distinguish between defiance and civil disobedience. Civil disobedience is a conscious, intentional, and public breaking of a law (Falcón y Tella 2004, 315). It is usually done collectively and with the expectation that the civilly disobedient will accept the legal sanctions against those actions. It is an act of law-breaking that is aimed at changing an unjust law where success counts as bringing about the change, and lack of change following civil disobedience tends to negate the efforts of disobedience. David Lefkowitz similarly defines civil disobedience as "deliberate disobedience to one or more laws of a state for the purpose of advocating a change to that state's laws or policies" (Lefkowitz 2007, 204). I am inclined to view the flag-burning that occurred during the Vietnam era as acts of defiance instead of civil disobedience;

flag-burners exhibited an in-your-face dramatization of their belief that the war was unjustified and malignant. Burning the American flag signified the scorn that the flag-burners felt toward an America that touts liberty and equality and yet perpetuates an unwinnable war. The objective of defiance, in this case, is not a change in law (as civil disobedience frequently aims at), but an expressive act to make a stand against American hypocrisy. In contrast to acts such as flag-burning, Lefkowitz emphasizes the quality of "suitably constrained" civil disobedience. It is one form of principled disobedience to the law (Lefkowitz 2007, 205). In such situations, individuals often need to act collectively in order to bring about a change while protecting the moral rights of all; collective action is often more effective at bringing about institutional changes.

But the difference between civil disobedience and defiance is not only about the ends at which they aim. Both defiance and civil disobedience affirm authoritative bodies' and oppressors' agency by treating them as agents, but the focus and attitudinal content of defiance are different from those of civil disobedience. Acts of civil disobedience make a moral claim on oppressors to recognize the humanity of the civilly disobedient. The civilly disobedient convey the message that the oppressors' own values require them to treat people differently from the way the people are being treated. Defiance speaks to norms as much as to persons, and it expresses that the oppressors' values are distorted or perverse. For example, when the Madres de la Plaza de Maya organized a movement in which their walking vigils marked their refusal to let the memory of their lost ones fade, they primarily were exhibiting defiance—of the authorities who demanded silence and acceptance from those whose loved ones were disappeared, and of norms of femaleness as willingly subordinate, forgiving, and suffering in silence. By calling out a social norm, defiers identify it as a product of oppressive structures that benefit the privileged while they burden the disenfranchised.

We may defy a norm for reasons of self-respect or with the aim of presenting a direct challenge. Consider an action during the inception of the Arab Spring of 2011. When 26-year-old Mohamed Bouazizi of Tunisia refused to turn over his fruits and vegetables cart to the police, he resisted or protested, but I would say he was not being defiant. However, when the policeman slapped him and publicly humiliated him, and he responded by setting himself on fire, he was acting defiantly. Bouazizi's act seemed to express that he would rather die than be subject to tyrannical rule any longer (although I would not say his defiant death is praiseworthy). Perhaps the most salient difference is that civil disobedience typically requires of the actors that they be willing to submit to the rule of law even if a punishing law is itself unjust.

Mahatma Gandhi and Martin Luther King led nonviolent protests in which their followers had to be ready and willing to accept the legal punishment. Neither civil disobedience nor defiance accurately can be described as sub-missive, but when leaders such as Gandhi or King emphasize not only accept-ance of legal punishment but also an attitude toward love of one's oppressors, their civil disobedience seems rather tame compared to defiance. Defiance, being "uncivil," is less tame, not just because it challenges or attacks cherished norms, but because it typically is unruly (more on this in Section 2.3.2).

The difference between civil disobedience and defiance is not always clear; it sometimes appears more like a family resemblance. Additionally, by marking a difference between the collective activities of civil disobedience and the apparently individual activity of defiance, I do not mean to suggest that defiance is individualistic. But with respect to those who are diagnosed with mental illnesses, defiant behavior is most often a dyadic relationship on the surface and a relationship between the individual sufferer and the insti-tutional norms of psychiatry on a deeper level. The nature of institutional structures within medicine makes patients' collective action difficult, if not impossible, to enact in the context of clinical encounters. However, collective action can *prepare* individuals for appropriate defiant behavior. The point is that, although defiant behavior is enacted by individuals instead of by groups, it is nevertheless relational, which relationality is significant when we arrive at later chapters.

2.3.2 Attitude and behavior

Defiance belongs with a cluster of attitudes and actions that include (but are not identical to) dissent, political (as contrasted with psychoanalytic) resist-ance, rebellion, and civil disobedience. A defiant action can be an "in your face" one; a defiant attitude usually comes across as openly and deliberately disrespectful (whether or not it means to be). In a refusal to bow to author-ity, the defiant person has the passion of anger (or indignation, or contempt) behind her. Defiance has less force and more limited scope than rebellion, but does not imply the "civilized" quality that dissent, resistance, and civil disobedience do. Those latter forms of protest typically are organized and pre-planned. Harking back to Cheng's comments on surviving imprisonment during the Cultural Revolution, I suggest that defiance *is* uncivilized, in the sense that socializing systems and hegemonic order enforce civility as defined by European-American values.

Defiance typically is also active rather than passive, and, for an act to be a defiant one, it must be more than merely refusing to participate. A person may refuse to pay income taxes because she does not want her tax money to be spent on the military or on the welfare of others, but this strikes me as more akin to the right to refuse treatment discussed in Chapter 1 than to defiance. My reasoning is that refusals to participate are more like acts of omission, and acts of omission are not emphatic or direct enough to function as a challenge to oppressive norms and practices. But even here, the concept of refusal does not neatly stay within tidy boundaries, and the active/passive distinction is analytic, not practical.

Consider the attitude of Traveling Thunder, a member of the Fort Belknap tribe, when Joseph Gone asked him under what conditions he would take a grandchild to a psychiatric clinic in Indian Health Services.

> "I would say that's kind of like taboo. You know, we don't do that. We never did do that" . . . That's like saying, you know, "What's the purpose of this reservation?" . . . The Whiteman can't see no purpose for it. But to the Indian people they say,
>
> "Well, this is my last stronghold", you know. "This is all I got left. I mean you took 99% of our land. You took our way of life. You wiped out all the buffalo . . . And then you'd rather slaughter the elk and the deer in the [National] Parks than give them to the Indian people on these reservations that are hungry . . ." I guess it's like a war, but they're not using bullets anymore . . . [Sigh] Like ethnic cleansing, I guess you could say. They want to wipe us out. Wipe the Indian reservations out so they could join the melting pot of the modern White society. And therefore the Indian problem will be gone forever . . . But they're using a more shrewder way than the old style of bullets. (Gone 2008, 381)

Traveling Thunder exhibits an attitude of defiance not only toward Western psychiatry but also toward the Whiteman. He is being disrespectful and uncivilized according to white, Western standards of civility. It is true that he responds to the First Nations' history of oppression with a refusal to participate, but his refusal is not passive; indeed, it is more than a mere refusal. Traveling Thunder's attitude and words stand directly, confrontationally, and in defiance of dominant norms in North American society. So although his "quiet" defiance might seem to undermine the idea of what constitutes defiance, I argue that he exhibits defiance that faces down direct authority.

To engage authority directly is important because it requires authoritative institutions or oppressors to acknowledge that their authority is being challenged. Traveling Thunder's quiet defiance in the face of white norms for mental health and civility counts as defiance, but quiet subterfuge in the face of dehumanization and subjugation is sometimes in accordance with cultural norms, while at other times it may be closer to a deficiency. Consider actions that are directly confrontational contrasted with passive-aggressive efforts at thwarting authority. Passive-aggressive behavior does not promote flourishing because it complicates our ability to get our needs met and for others to take seriously our needs and expectations. Marcia Linehan's description of active passivity is the sort of thing I have in mind, where the person is actively seeking help from others but not engaging in problem-solving herself (1993, 78). Linehan distinguishes active passivity from learned helplessness, the latter expressing that the person has given up on seeking help from others. It's not so much that active passivity is ineffective as that its indirectness takes the parties involved on a circuitous and unclear path toward problem-solving. Furthermore, in active passivity, the person's solicitations for help may be experienced by others as demanding or clinging, and a vicious cycle of demandingness/invalidation between the parties is begun. Active passivity, or passive-aggressive behavior, fall short of good defiance because they undermine the agent's communicative power and hinder her ability to express self-worth. Linehan notes that active passivity occurs more in women than men, and she cites evidence that women are encouraged to use indirect and sometimes helpless modes in problem-solving (1993, 80). This is where one form of the language of resistance can be found, the kind discussed in Chapter 1. This form of resistance is not political in nature but, instead, is rooted in intrapsychic beliefs and often unconscious attitudes. In order to be defiant, then, we must directly and openly stand against and, often, engage authoritative power in the form of norms, persons, or policies.

Still, a lot of behavior we call "defiant" is not defiant, by my definition. Consider the hackers' forums that "cohere" to form temporary online groups engaged in planning and executing a significant disruption in the functioning of a major corporation or institution. The most well-known and effective hackers, as of this writing, are individuals who identify themselves as "Anonymous." While the operations and computer savvy of Anonymous are far too complex and detailed to be explained here (see Olson 2012), Anonymous itself has a motive and rationale behind their activities that typically aims at retribution—for example, hacking into the website of the Church of Scientology with the objective of causing massive disruption in its functioning because it suppressed information (a video of Tom Cruise that was potentially damaging to the reputation and status of the Church of Scientology). To be sure, Anonymous is out to have fun, but it also self-identifies as defying authority in its suppression of freedom of speech. Such activities, as I see them, in the main are not defiant even though they flaunt the power of institutions' and corporations' ability to suppress and control the dissemination of information. I say this because Anonymous's aim primarily is to seek retribution, do damage, and cause disruption.

As I have argued, defiance can challenge people's relationship to power and authority and to social norms that tend to preserve the status quo. It is precisely because differences in power can impede the flourishing of those living under or with adverse conditions that we need virtues such as defiance that specifically target the injustices and harms that the disenfranchised experience. This is not to say that any and all uses of power are illegitimate or that any person in a position of authoritative power necessarily impedes the flourishing of the disadvantaged or less powerful. Many psychiatrists can and do use their position of power and expertise to help patients, and sometimes patients' defiance can interfere with what is good for them in the long run. Psychiatrists can use their power to help patients through what may be troublesome defiant behavior. However, as I argue in later chapters, psychiatrists' desire to give good and appropriate guidance to patients often is complicated by nosological, epistemological, and ethical norms and assumptions. One of the central aims of this book is to uncover such norms and assumptions so that psychiatrists can diagnose and treat people more appropriately and accurately. The point here is that, as Tessman says, "having to develop virtues that are disconnected from flourishing can be understood as a real deprivation created by oppressive conditions" (Tessman 2005, 49). Structures within society seem to insist that the marginalized, oppressed and, even to some degree, the mentally disabled, learn (or at least pretend to learn) the values of civility, cooperation, and so on, even on pain of developing damaged characters. (Think of the "good patient" role and the expectation of compliance I discussed in Chapter 1.) Tessman calls such virtues "burdened." I argue that there are three ways in which to understand defiance in light of Tessman's work:

1. defiance can be an unburdened virtue;
2. defiance can be a burdened virtue itself; and
3. defiance can be either
   a. a vice; or
   b. a symptom of mental disorder.

In the case of (2), defiance can just replace one burdened virtue with another, and in (3), defiance is not a virtue at all. I present these possibilities as analytically distinct, but in everyday life, they may overlap and come in gradations. This book emphasizes (1), but in order to make sense of defiance as an unburdened virtue, I next explain what burdened virtues are. Chapter 3 goes into more detail on this matter.

2.4 **Burdened virtues**

Aristotle's theory of flourishing, or well-being, requires that the path by which people can achieve *eudaimonia*, or flourishing, is through cultivating virtues. Virtues such as justice, truth-telling, friendship, and courage are good qualities of character for people to have. But Aristotle presents a world in which the background conditions for living well are ideal. Although Aristotle pays attention to power differentials, he naturalizes those differences and, instead of worrying about the negative consequences that being subordinated or subjugated entails, he endorses them. The actual world, however, is one where many (if not most) people live under adverse background conditions, including "the more wretched conditions present under some forms of oppression," as Lisa Tessman says (2009, 48). Thus, in our non-ideal world, even being virtuous is insufficient for living well. An Aristotelian conception of *eudaimonia* functions as an ideology that, while claiming an integral connection between being virtuous and flourishing, is unattainable for many, if not most, people. But Tessman does believe that, even in a non-ideal world, "a trait may still qualify as a virtue when it is detrimental to an agent's well-being" (Tessman 2005, 52). Later chapters provide further details of this view. Her approach is to retain the concept of flourishing even when it is unattainable, while still holding that some virtues are worthy of cultivating and exercising and that flourishing is a worthy value. Tessman calls virtues that are severed from flourishing "burdened virtues." This characterization allows us to mark them as constitutive of the moral damage caused by trying to live out norms and expectations that keep those who live under adverse conditions occupying an inferior position.

Burdened virtues are those that burden the moral efforts of the oppressed because of harm done to them. Tessman draws upon Claudia Card's idea of "moral damage," a way to characterize the harms done to subordinated people when they are not able to exercise the virtues (Tessman 2005, 51; cf. Card 1990). Tessman argues that, under oppressive conditions, many people's reasoning is affected by a distorted view of acting well or virtuously and that people's desires are also distorted by a need to adapt to relations of domination and subordination (Tessman 2005, 50). I draw upon Tessman's proposal for a non-ideal eudaimonism in offering a virtue ethics that is practical and realistic for those living in adverse conditions. By "adverse conditions," I mean those who live with mental illnesses, but also those colonized, racialized, and gendered as inferior, subordinate and, even, erased (Lugones 2007; Hale 2009). "Non-ideal ethical theory must recognize flourishing as being out of reach under some conditions of oppression and must contribute to understanding moral life given this fact" (Tessman 2009, 48).

In an ideal world, (privileged) moral agents are granted a capacity for practical reasoning and the ability for desires to be governed by correct reasoning. Aristotle presents moral agents (that is, the elite citizens of Greece) as interdependent in the sense that what is good for oneself also contributes to the good of others (his idea that "a friend is another self" is an example of this idea). But, as Tessman points out, such an assumption elides the real-world conditions where interdependence is replaced by relations of domination and subordination (2009, 49). She argues that

> In a non-idealized eudaimonistic virtue ethics, one will have to assume that flourishing will be largely unattainable, in part because of moral damage, that is, damage to the virtues, and in part because of adverse external conditions. (Tessman 2009, 51)

Burdened virtues, then, are ones that, while being "virtues" in a decontextualized sense, fail to contribute to the oppressed person's ability to live a flourishing life. That is, such virtues contribute to the workings of society *as a whole*, but do not enhance the experience or life of the particular person exhibiting the virtue.

Tessman starts from the empirical claim that oppression interferes with flourishing. For example, she discusses the (virtually worldwide) norm that women be self-sacrificing in service to their families, and argues that the cost of living out this norm is that women "are unable to pursue their own interests as long as their interests conflict with that of others" (2005, 67). Systems of oppression create dispositions that are subjugated, yet the subjugated self may long for liberation. The conflict between the subjugated disposition and liberatory beliefs is not amenable to mere "bootstrapping." As Tessman puts it, "the special problem of figuring out how to resist oppression creates the question of how to change the vices in the oppressed that may contribute to their own suffering and that may prevent them from (successfully) pursuing liberation" (2005, 19). It is in this spirit that I propose the virtue of defiance.

A shift in focus to oppressive structures instead of focusing on individual character flaws does not detract from the concern that some "virtues" of the oppressed do not contribute to flourishing and may, in fact, do harm to the oppressed. Tessman suggests that, in thinking about virtues under oppressive conditions, we should ask,

> [D]oes the character trait help its bearer to engage in liberatory struggles, the purpose of which is to eventually enable a good life for all? Or, alternatively, one might ponder, does the character trait help its bearer to live well now (or to contribute to others' living well now,) in the context of continuing oppression . . .? (Tessman 2005, 52)

In this passage, Tessman is offering two important tests for determining whether a character trait will contribute to experiences of liberation for those living under oppressive conditions, each of which test has its place. One test is that of being able to survive the dehumanization and humiliation of being oppressed, and the other is that of furthering the aims of the oppressed for liberation from their oppressors.

I am concerned about harms as they intersect with people whose history and socioeconomic status places them at a disadvantage—in particular, those with mental distress. As Tessman's work on burdened virtues suggests, defiance does not necessarily release one from the damages of living within oppressive or disadvantaged conditions (Tessman 2005, 108). For all of us, our lives are embedded in the social and historical context of our lived conditions; our experiences are informed by cultural values, contested affiliations, assumptions about rationality and mental health, and epistemic, legal, moral, and linguistic norms. People who have (or may have) mental illnesses are no exception, and so we are likely to misunderstand acts of defiance if we decontextualize them or try to interact with people as if they are mere individuals with a personal, family, and medical history that is supposed to inform treatment in the abstract. In addition, some of the people who come from adverse backgrounds also experience encounters with psychiatrists that further exacerbate distrust, a sense of unfair treatment, and moral harm done. The intersection of living under oppressive conditions (such as poverty, racialization, and trans- and homophobia) and living under adverse conditions (such as mental illness) is complicated by the ways that the diagnosis of mental illness historically has been used to contain and further subjugate the already oppressed (cf. Metzl 2009; Ussher 2011). Not all those who are classified as mentally ill have lived under oppressive conditions, but when considering the endemic existence of racialized, classed, and gendered people, it is likely that many have. Furthermore, it is undeniable that the institution of psychiatry has not always been neutral and benign in its determinations, such that even privileged classes of people may experience their encounters with psychiatry as oppressive. This is not to imply that individual psychiatrists intentionally are doing harm to people, but that the ideology and status of psychiatry as an institution can be oppressive. (Chapter 6 addresses this claim in detail and explains how psychiatrists can use the ideas in this book—in particular, by developing the virtue of giving uptake to defiant people.) The significance of these points is that, sometimes, people who are behaving in ways that defy social norms are taken up as mentally ill when they should not be, and that even those with mental illnesses may be defiant appropriately. But under what circumstances, then, is defiance a virtue, instead of just a tactical behavior (perhaps an excessive one) or an expression like "ouch"?

Loosely placing defiance within a non-ideal eudaimonistic virtue ethics, I suggest that defiance is one of the dispositions worth cultivating because, when expressed within the mean, defiance can contribute to well-being. To be defiant is to express a challenge to authoritative norms, be it through atti-tude, speech, other communication, behavior, and, in the case of Traveling Thunder, one of long-standing opposition to overwhelming colonialist pres-sure to buckle to dominant norms. It is not "civilized" or domesticated.[1] It is often, but not always, loud, angry, and "in your face." But it makes itself known and felt as a deliberate stand against injustice, oppression, or other forms of unfairness, both interpersonal and structural. It contributes to well-being because it declares one's self-respect and self-worth in the face of pressure to submit, to comply, to accept.

A disposition to be defiant is a tendency to be able to recognize a situation that calls for defiance and the readiness to act when such a situation arises. In other words, this is the dispositional mean or intermediate condition. Like other virtues, defiance has extremes. Adopting an Aristotelian framework, the deficiency would be submission of, or resignation to, the norms that struc-ture one's social position as subordinate and inferior. I consider the deficiency to be paradigmatic of defiance as a burdened virtue. I do not mean that a dispositional deficiency is always a burdened virtue, but that it often follows along lines of social structures where burdened virtues attach to disadvan-taged people and those who live in adverse conditions. The excess would be physical violence, aggression within other subordinate groups (horizontal violence), and law-breaking that serves one's own interests at the expense of others within one's own community and other groups with whom one shares commonalities of oppression. Being defiant is not a mere knee-jerk reac-tion: the person who acts defiantly has done some conscious (perhaps even consciousness-raising), psychological, and, often, political background pre-paratory work. She or he may have engaged in self-reflection. She or he may have been part of a circle of people who, together, interrogated various ways of interpreting their worlds. Defiance as a character trait has a reasoning quality as well, but it does not require rationality as it is deployed within master nar-ratives (see Box 2.1 for an explanation of master narratives).

The point is that defiance as a virtue is not "irrational," although it is often interpreted that way within the workplace, educational systems, and psych-iatry. Carving out the ways in which defiance is reasonable is difficult because it goes against the grain of ontological commitments to the ideal of the civi-lized, autonomous, and self-sufficient rational beings we "mostly are." The expression of defiance in psychiatric settings challenges the binary of reason-ing well or poorly and the binary of "mental health" versus "mental illness." Such challenges are important especially in the domain of psychiatry where a central part (but not the only part) of conceptualizing mental disorder and dysfunction is through flawed reasoning. My theory of defiance strikes at the

Box 2.1 Master narratives

Master narratives organize societal beliefs, values, and aims in an apparently logical fashion. They are little questioned; instead, they are unwittingly taken as true, reproducing dominant themes of everyday living and marginalizing the voices that are less coherently woven in or that lack fitness.

> Master narratives are often archetypal, consisting of stock plots and readily recognizable character types, and we use them not only to make sense of our experience . . . but also to justify what we do. . . . As the repositories of common norms, master narratives exercise a certain authority over our moral imaginations and play a role in informing our moral intuitions. (Nelson 2001, 6)

Master narratives, because they emerge and are sustained by dominant groups and their ideologies, beliefs, and values, construct identities of subgroups that serve the dominant groups' purposes. Sometimes, for example with racialized groups, the stories told about the "nature" of the subgroup cast them as "undeserving of moral consideration, or as morally intolerable" (Nelson 2001, 107). If members of the subgroup do not accept the norms of the dominant group (for instance, they resist or defy), they are cast as unruly in morally degrading (or pathologizing, I would add) terms (Nelson 2001, 107). Master narratives, such as ones that entail the domain of rationality, make it difficult to interpret defiant behavior accurately.

heart of norms of mental health and rationality through an investigation into the history and legacy of diagnosing disorders in psychiatry when people are strange, unruly and, by dominant cultural standards, incomprehensibly putting themselves at risk—what psychiatrists might identify as threatening people's very ability to flourish or live well. Given structural power differences in their historical and ongoing manifestations, together with a history of using psychiatric means to contain and control those deemed dangerous to colonial and hegemonic powers, our very conception of "good" and "bad" mental health, and "good" and "bad" reasoning may be distorted. An examination of defiance gives us a glimmer of a different conception. Defiant logics stand ambiguously at the boundaries of what it even means to "reason well" and it is in our interests to subvert and to play with the margins between reasoning well and badly. Nevertheless, defiant behavior can be excessive; it can arise as a response to burdened virtues; and it can be a symptom of mental disorder. Section 2.5 provides some cases of the extremes.

2.5 **Examples of extremes**

Drawing on Tessman's work, in which she argues that gendered and racial-ized systems of character formation create people who are afraid to fight back (Tessman 2005, 38), I suggest that defiance as a character trait can "enable one to resist oppression . . . or to flourish as one would if one had already escaped oppression" (Tessman 2005, 23). Behaving defiantly, then, one may aim for a relatively modest goal of asserting one's separateness from oppressive norms, but one can also hold a broader goal of agitating for social change. That is, defiance, properly understood, is liberatory for one's character, and liberating oneself from damaging and oppressive norms, expectations, and conditions will sometimes contribute to one's flourishing. It may be liberatory in that it affirms the defier's self-respect while pointing to norms that claim to contrib-ute to social well-being but instead are suspected of thwarting and frustrating the development of parts of society and community.

As with other virtues, defiance has extremes and a mean. The deficiency would seem to be submission, fatalism, hopeless, or subservience; the excess is something like random lawlessness, continually in-your-face actions, or belligerence. I am particularly concerned with ways in which acquiescence to authority is inculcated in members of minority and disadvantaged groups and considered to be a benign process of socialization into proper civility. On this analysis, those who are successfully socialized are more likely than not to have a deficiency of defiance.

Defiance is a virtue that, in the right contexts and within the mean, can help correct for moral damage. For example, consider the burdened virtue of being submissive. Curtis Sittenfeld describes how female submissiveness insidiously warps girls' lives. She writes,

> In fifth grade, you can run faster than any other girl in your class . . . At recess, you're the foursquare queen. You slam the red rubber ball onto your three opponents' patches of pavement, and you gloat when they get disqualified . . . Once, after [the teacher has] rung the bell to call you inside, you pass her, your body still tense and excited, your face flushed. She says in a low voice, a voice that sounds more like the one she uses with adults and not with the other children in your class, "Anna, aren't you being just a bit vicious?" The next time you're playing, you fumble and let the ball slide beyond the thin white lines that serve as boundaries. (Sittenfeld 2001, 3)

Sittenfeld explains the insidious ways in which the socialization of females frames physical skill and energy as a vice of aggression; what, for Sittenfeld, is a vice, would count as a virtue for the boys. Sittenfeld understood that, to be a "good" girl, she could not be a successful athlete. This outcome is particu-larly worrisome in light of research by Gilligan and Brown on adolescent girls' loss of voices (cf. Gilligan and Brown 1992). Sittenfeld, like millions of girls globally, is discouraged from engaging in activities that boys are rewarded for doing. If Sittenfeld insists on playing sports her way, she will probably be judged as defiant and the teacher will come down harder (and less privately) on her. To earn her teacher's praise, she must forgo her personal style and put on a performance of femininity. In my view, the virtue of femininity is a burdened virtue à la Tessman, and if Sittenfeld were able to openly resist and refute the teacher's authority, she could retain some self-respect and joy in her life. As it stands, Sittenfeld describes the situation of many girls who have a deficiency of defiance.

Consider the next example of a young woman whose behavior is judged to be defiant.

> In the late Middle Ages, [white] 22-year-old Anna Büschler was banished from her widowed father's home for having taken not one, but two lovers. She took him to court, charging him with abandonment. When he later captured her, her father—the Bürgermeister—chained her to a kitchen table for six months, until a servant helped her escape. He disinherited her. She sued him again. In fact, Büschler spent the next 30 years in litigation against her father. (Ozment 1996)

Although punished severely, Büschler exhibited a kind of feisty integrity, and I offer her story as an example of someone who has a disposition to be defiant. Büschler surely was defiant—of the norms for proper womanliness in the Middle Ages, and of the proper place of a daughter under patriarchy. Was it good that she was defiant? Well, "good for whom?" It certainly was not good in terms of social harmony, as it was conceived in the Middle Ages, that a woman open defied such norms. But it may have been good for other women, who later benefited from Büschler's lawsuits against her father. This example underscores the importance of understanding defiant behavior as it occurs in local situations and in terms of local norms. Defiance is context-dependent but not relative, as I stated in Section 2.2. Additionally, if one's protest is likely to lead to persecution, and unlikely to bring about relief, then the question arises as to what the point even of good defiance would be. I return to this question in Chapter 3, where I set out Tessman's different ways of conceptualizing virtuous traits, and then in Chapter 4, where I discuss cultural factors in interpreting defiant behavior in children. In brief, however, I suggest that Büschler's behavior was not excessive, although it still may have been burdened.

As additional fodder, I also call readers' attention to the many examples from fiction where the main female character has her defiant attitude toward the status quo stamped out of her until she forfeits her agency through death. I have in mind George Eliott's *Mill on the Floss* (Maggie), Gustav Flaubert's *Madame Bovary* (Emma), Leo Tolstoy's *Anna Karenina* (Anna), and Edith

Wharton's *House of Mirth* (Lily Bart). In each of these novels, the female figure defies social norms—especially gender norms—and suffers such that her life is no longer worth living. Such novels educate readers into the dangers of defiance by first engaging our sympathies with the stifled female and then our sense of tragic loss at her death. Readers may be outraged at the turn the heroine's life has taken, but many readers also absorb the message that, if only she hadn't taken things so far, she could have avoided a senseless death. Such novels function as a warning against defying cultural and gender norms.

The next example concerns political leadership. There are many instances of excessive or bad defiance to be found in the political domain, so I have chosen one from American politics. George W. Bush, former president of the United States, acted in defiance of the law with his secret policy on domestic spying without a warrant, and in defiance of the Geneva Convention by signing a bill that allows intelligence officers to interrogate suspects with force. Bush seems to have a disposition to be defiant, but his defiance fails to be virtuous because he uses his position of power to violate people's human rights. Of course, one could argue that, as a world leader, he had a responsibility to defy norms that would prevent the security of the nation. So, this sort of case is difficult. The problem with Bush's defiance is that it perpetuates unjust inequalities and structurally unfair treatment. The consequences of being defiant depend on where one is located within social structures, and disciplining stratifies people: those with privilege become more powerful (and sometimes more arrogant) by their privilege being normalized. But the excessively privileged are outliers: they have so much power that they can be defiant of, say, constitutional law. Then defiance functions as an *exercise* of power. Defiance as an excessive and dispositional use of power (whether or not that power is legitimate) is a vice—first of all because it undermines flourishing; and, secondly, as in the case of Bush, because it is an illegitimate exercise of power. Furthermore, defiance as a vice impedes—prohibits, even—another virtue: justice. On the other hand, it is possible for a person in a position of power to use that authority to liberate or further others' flourishing. That is, people can exercise power in a legitimate and constructive way, as many (perhaps most) psychiatrists do.

When one in authority uses one's power in an illegitimate way, one may open up the possibility for others to respond defiantly to that use of authoritative power. The next investigation into possible excesses of defiance returns our attention to those with relatively less power and emphasizes the point that the success of liberatory defiance is constrained by the cultural context in which oppression and defiance are mediated. Christina Doza's English teacher had been sexually harassing her, so she wrote a crude comment about him in her zine. The teacher got hold of a copy of the zine and he asked Doza to apologize.

> I tell him the comment was only the truth, and we both know it, and I'm not going to sit here and play psychological warfare with him. I tell him he's a piece of shit, and I'll apologize the day hell freezes over. I tell him he better think again if he thinks he can tell me what to do with my zine. (Doza 2001, 43)

Like Büschler, Doza shows feisty integrity. But did she tell him off "in the right way"? The answer depends on how we understand the mean in relation to defiance. As discussed in Section 2.3, defiance is not one of the "civilized" virtues. So, respectfully and civilly telling off her English teacher would not count as defiance; it is too acquiescent of the teacher's authoritative position given his sexual harassment. Was Doza's response excessive? I am inclined to say that it was not excessive, given that the teacher was intrusive not only intellectually but also sexually. Still, her abusive language and communications render a clear judgment difficult to make concerning the appropriateness of her defiant behavior. Just how untamed can defiance be and still be considered within the mean? I consider this question in more detail in later chapters, but for now I emphasize the point that Doza's defiance must be understood in the context of her teacher's sexual harassment. Given the type of infraction and the harm done by sexual harassment, when a person is sexually harassed, a greater degree of defiance is reasonable.

An additional question that arises when we consider Doza's situation is whether her defiance is wise. This is an important question, since virtues are supposed to reflect reason. The answer would seem to depend on how we understand doing a virtuous thing "for the right end." For defiance to be a virtue, the object of the defiance must be some oppressive norm, condition or, even, a person; the aim is either liberatory for the subordinated person or for other subordinated peoples or, as Tessman says, it enables them to live well now—for example, by claiming self-respect or making clear to oneself and others that one is not acquiescing in oppressive structures. Doza's defiance may be similar to the anarchic idea of creating Temporary Autonomous Zones, the "idea of acting freely in a repressive context, of acting "as if one lived in a free society," creating zones of increasing freedom and viewing these as the proper end of oppositional action" (Goldfarb 1998, 89–90). By being defiant, Doza preserves her integrity and outrightly rejects her English teacher's claims to subordinate her, affirming, at least temporarily, her autonomy from him—important ends, I would think. Still, it is not clear that the long-term consequences of defiance won't compromise her chances at flourishing. I return to the topic of flourishing in Chapter 3.

Taking a step back, let's consider what it means to orient questions of the virtue of Doza's actions to that of practical reasoning. Asking whether Doza's defiance was wise is, on my analysis, to expect defiance to be tamed enough to reflect reason—certainly the Aristotelian way to think about virtues—but it also corrals Doza within disciplinary structures at a point where she is trying to defy them. On the other hand, without reason, her defiance may be self-defeating, such as if her actions give others (apparent) justification to oppress her further, or diagnose her as "mad." The topic of norms for practical reasoning by which to evaluate defiant behavior is covered in Chapter 5.

The last case for discussion in this chapter is one that I take to be a fairly clear example of an excess of defiance that arises out of moral damage. The film *Ladybird, Ladybird* (1994), based on a true story, depicts Maggie, a working-class mother of four children by four different fathers, as suspicious and distrustful of the social welfare system in Britain and frustrated in her ability to care for her children. We meet Maggie after her four children have been removed from her home after a fire broke out one night while she was working and jeopardized the lives of her children. When Maggie gets pregnant by a Peruvian illegal immigrant named Jorge, welfare workers take this child away as well, on the grounds that she is not a fit mother—decisions that, according to the film, are tainted by classism and racism. The heartbreaking story unfolds of a mother in the clutches of social workers, whose hope of regaining custody of her children rests on her ability to satisfy the court that she has her children's best interests in mind and can protect them from harm. Maggie, unfortunately, cannot perform as the court, social services, her lawyer, and even her new partner, require of her. At sea since childhood in a child welfare system that repeatedly has failed her, Maggie is unwilling or unable to sit quietly during social worker visits or at trial. She defiantly shouts out of turn in court, tells off the social workers whose home visits are designed to establish Maggie's maturity and trustworthiness, and throws off Jorge's consoling caresses in front of others to see. Interpreting her behavior through lenses of class privilege and racial bias, the court deems her to be of limited intelligence and an unfit mother. The long-term consequence of her defiance of social and extra-legal norms is the removal of even more of her children from her home. The courts' biases in making these decisions compromised their epistemic and moral responsibilities to evaluate Maggie's behavior through just lens. Nevertheless, I am inclined to think that Maggie's defiant behavior was excessive because it failed to further her interests, seemed to miss the mark of self-respecting demeanor, and seemed to be (perhaps unconsciously) driven by unregulated emotion. To the extent that defiance requires an accurate reading of the situation such that the defier can apply the mean while retaining her sense of challenge to the social and gender norms, Maggie seemed unable either to assess situations accurately or to control her outbursts to the degree that she can turn them to her advantage. The "mad or bad" dichotomy also seems to be at play here. The court, after looking at the records and listening to testimony, deemed Maggie to be "bad"—(i.e., a bad mother)—instead of "mad" (as in having a mental disorder). I interpret Maggie's defiance to have arisen out of moral damage. That is, I do not think it is symptomatic of a personality disorder, as the court seems to think. Maggie might be said to have a character flaw, but one that must be understood as shaped and habituated by her adverse life experiences and her current crisis of facing the permanent loss of her children.

Sometimes, however, defiant behavior is neither a vice nor a virtue but, instead, is a symptom of mental disorder. This latter possibility corresponds to 3b in Section 2.3.2. Perhaps the clearest example of 3b is that of Grayson,[2] who is brought into the emergency room because his floridly psychotic state causes him to be violent and aggressive. Grayson responds to any attempt by anyone to subdue him—whether or not that person is in an authoritative role—by becoming more violent and aggressive toward others. Grayson does not seem to be reasoning at all but, instead, seems to be acting impulsively or instinctively. His behavior is defiant, but it is defiance that is caused by, and arises out of, a psychotic state and, therefore, cannot be considered either a vice or a virtue. In general, then, a person has the virtue of defiance when: a) he or she shows a readiness to be defiant when situations call for it; b) he or she employs *phronesis* adequately and finds the intermediate condition between the extremes; c) he or she exhibits attitudes, feelings, and behaviors consistent with defiance; and d) he or she is able to evaluate consequences and to aim for flourishing.

2.6 **Conclusion**

I conclude this chapter with some clarifying remarks about my theory of defiance. An obvious concern about advocating defiance is that individual acts of defiance may be met with the full force of oppressive and abusive powers, and defiant groups may be read as excessive and subsequently be suppressed. Collective defiance may, therefore, require considerable strategic planning and deliberation in order for members' defiant voices to be heard without evoking suppression. Social movements involving collective defiance often eventually find that the "mean" amounts to "moderation." As I argued, as defiance moves toward the reflective, it becomes tamed. Defiance becomes domesticated.

Here we see the struggle between radical movements that press against boundaries and a felt need for members of those movements to tone themselves down so as to be more "effective." The problem is precisely this: there is a place for socialization and civilized behavior, but it sometimes can undermine the possibility of transformation. So the apparent excess of the moment is important to keep because, for defiance to be genuinely empowering, it tends to require social organizing and, hence, more reflective strategizing. Yet, as it moves to the collective and reflective, it becomes "tamed" and hence less recognizable as defiance.

The institutionalization of maintaining social order sometimes requires punishing and diagnosing. But keeping people in line has an inherent structure that props up an imbalance of power, and that imbalance of power can be abusive. Social structures must be maintained. Some people are in the business of ensuring that disciplinary structures are enforced, and others are recruited to maintain them—for example, as in U.S. military policy regarding "enhanced interrogation techniques" of prisoners at Abu Graib, at one level, and the guards and medical military personnel who performed the actual torture, at another level. Others become victims of the disciplines of oppression. The mechanics of society can be numbing, and people can become so comfortable living within status quo ideologies that we no longer think critically about the body politic. Defiance infuses into the body politic an element of raw human will. And, while raw human will seems to be a vital quality of defiance when expressed by the disenfranchised, it also is a quality expressed by governments, educational systems, prisons, and corporations. Whether it is individual or structural, defiance can jostle the social body to wakefulness and, potentially, to broader social criticism. When the disenfranchised express defiance, then, they can provide a check on abuses of power—provided power structures have fissures enough for defiance to erupt.

Burdened virtues, such as those Tessman so richly analyzes, may not be ones we need in an egalitarian and emancipatory future. I do not entertain utopian ideals. Nevertheless, as I claimed in Section 2.3.2, sometimes defiance is an unburdened virtue. I develop Tessman's theory of burdened virtues in Chapter Three. Here, I describe the case of my daughter Katrina, whose photographs in her workplace only show her with another woman of her own age. Katrina flaunts norms of familial depictions in her workplace, and she does so proudly and without regret or residual conflict. When people ask if the other woman is her sister, she answers that it is her wife, knowing that most listeners will be uncomfortable or even judgmental. She understands that there may be consequences for her actions—that there are always consequences of one's actions—and she accepts them because living openly as a lesbian is constitutive of living well. I will add, but not argue for, the claim that defying heteronormativity is not just subjectively constitutive of living well but is objectively so. I consider Katrina's defiance of these norms and with these features to be an unburdened virtue. It is important to note, however, that Katrina is able to be comfortable in the workplace when she defies heterosexual familial norms because anti-discrimination laws protect such expressions as her photographs address.

I expect defiance as a virtue to stay around. Hegemonic and oppressive structures, and distorted interpersonal relationships, may continue, and defiance can function as a check on those in authority and with (access to) power so that power does not remain oppressive. Additionally, complacency is a risk with even the best societies, and defiance is a way to disrupt the false consciousness of prevailing ideologies.

This chapter has focused almost entirely on social politics as I presented my theory of defiance. The next chapter focuses on psychiatric cases and questions of flourishing.

Chapter 3

Good defiance and flourishing

Passions, burdened virtues, and standards of flourishing are central topics of Chapter 3. In the last chapter, I stated that defiance sometimes is an unburdened virtue. The reason is that it is allows us to aim toward flourishing even when the bar may be set impossibly high. In this chapter, I examine the relationship between defiance and flourishing by analyzing three cases and unpacking some of the epistemic and ontological assumptions that undergird our naïve ideas about flourishing. By drawing on more informed theory, I explain how I would evaluate three cases of defiant behavior.

3.1 Schizophrenia

Henry Cockburn was diagnosed with schizophrenia when he was twenty years old. Henry had visions but did not believe he was ill; he considered himself to be having "magical experiences." Because he did not believe he was mentally ill, he kept running away from hospitals:

> Most of the time, I was spitting out my medication. I wanted to run away because running away had become crucial to my life.... I went by the railway line and took my shoes off. The tree talked to me in a sort of Shakespearean rhyme:
>
> > You must not act the knave
> > When others rant and rave.
>
> I asked about the monsoon that the tree I had talked to nearly two years earlier had predicted, and it said, "The towers will be surrounded by water."
>
> . . .
>
> I took my clothes off and felt cold. I walked by the train tracks until I stepped on a thorn and fell over just seconds before a train raced past. I was lucky that I wasn't seen. If someone had seen a naked man walking by the train tracks, they would have told the police. (Cockburn and Cockburn 2011, 121–2)

Henry is noncompliant in a number of ways. Medically, he might be considered noncompliant because he runs away from the hospital, only pretends to take his meds, and, we might say, because he takes off all his clothes when it is so cold out. We might also count that last type of noncompliance as social noncompliance, in that it knowingly defies the norms for appearance in public. But Henry can also be viewed as defiant: his actions of escaping hospital, pretending to take medications, and flaunting norms for behavior in public all fit the characteristics of defiance I described in Chapter 2. The question I am considering here is how to think about Henry's defiance: is it good or bad? And from whose perspective? Is there a proper perspective to take when thinking about defiance, or is it subjective? Additionally, perhaps those categories of "good" and "bad" do not fit defiance in the case of Henry and others afflicted with severe mental illnesses. If defiance is supposed to contribute to a degree of flourishing, it might be the case that some patients' behavior should not be characterized as defiance at all. Can we see Henry's behavior as contributory to his flourishing?

The naïve response is to say that, of course, Henry is not flourishing: he practically kills himself with behavior caused by schizophrenia. But from Henry's perspective, his doctors, his hospital stays, his medications, and his overall diagnosis as schizophrenic was a gross misunderstanding of his experiences. His distrust of psychiatrists' (and his family's) interpretation of his needs and desires led him to believe he was being unjustly confined and controlled. This is Henry's subjective understanding of the phenomena that others viewed as symptoms—and, although the patient's subjective interpretation of his life experiences are crucial to take into consideration, they do not *settle* questions about the reasonableness of defiance. Those answers must be sought in a balance between a subjective and an objective epistemic and ethical space. The development of this point is taken up in Chapter 5, where I set out some features of practical reasoning and analyze how they might apply to Henry's behavior. Here, I give an account of flourishing and show how it is tied to normative notions of reasoning. I argue that a certain way of understanding reasoning is related to the aim of flourishing and suggest that the exercise of some kind of reasoning is important even when flourishing cannot be actualized under adverse conditions. I suggest that a more nuanced understanding of flourishing and reasoning allow a more accurate evaluation of Henry's and other cases of defiance.

3.2 **Flourishing**

As I argued in Chapter 2, flourishing may be an unrealistic ideal not only for those living under oppressive circumstances, but also for many of those living under adverse conditions such as the presence of mental disabilities. Yet, as Tessman and I argue, it does not follow that we should overthrow the aim of flourishing; Thomas Pogge, Martha Nussbaum, and other scholars note that identifying criteria for justice presupposes a concept of human flourishing (Pogge 1999; Nussbaum 2000, 1992). The challenge is to understand it properly. In Section 3.2.1, I return to Aristotle's ideal account of flourishing. Because I situate defiance in an Aristotelian virtue ethics framework, I need to distinguish his essentialist account of flourishing from my own account. I then turn to the idea of non-ideal flourishing to apply it to questions about the relationship between flourishing and defiance. Flourishing, liberation from oppression and other struggles in living, and defiance thus form a cluster of concepts that loosen academic as well as popular accounts of reasoning and rationality. This framework positions me to propose fresh ways of thinking about particular cases.

3.2.1 Aristotle on flourishing

First, let's get a clearer idea of what Aristotle has in mind by living a flourishing life. Aristotle's *eudaimonia* is integrally bound up in an idea that all living entities have a function that is essential to their nature (Aristotle 2000, NE Bk I). To fulfill their function well, organisms need to become excellent representatives of their species. Humans have a unique, species-specific function: to use reason excellently in order to become virtuous in character and intellect (Aristotle 2000, NE 1098a7–15). That is, the virtues are necessary in order to live a flourishing life. Human flourishing is objectively choiceworthy. Thus, it is ontological; it is a state of being, not merely an experience or a subjective feeling. On Aristotle's virtue theory, the ontological status of flourishing is tied to ideas about the species-specific characteristics of humanness. That is, being human is a particular, unique kind of entity, one whose capabilities and potentialities are what make it possible for us as a kind to unfold and become the same kind of thing from generation to generation—what Montgomery Furth calls "resistance to migration" (Furth 1988). In Aristotle's metaphysics of substance, "If *man* and *wolf* are (distinct) substantial kinds, THEN they include migration-barriers such that one and the same object cannot be earlier a man and later a wolf" (Furth 1988, 56; emphasis in original). The anti-migration law thus preserves the essence of a given species over time.

Now, it is true that Aristotle is not, strictly speaking, a universalist when it comes to the application of virtue theory. Because human flourishing is not merely abstract and generic, and because it requires activity—the activity of individuals who are always situated and located in a particular culture, time, and ethos—human flourishing is agent-specific. Aristotle can be misunderstood in this respect, because he defines virtue as "a state that decides, consisting in a mean, *the mean relative to us*, which is defined by reference to reason, that is to say, to the reason by reference to which the prudent person would define it" (Aristotle 2000, 1107a; emphasis added). What he means by this is not that virtues are relative or subjective, but that they are *contextual*. He offers a heuristic device known as the Doctrine of the Mean:

> We can be afraid, for instance, or be confident, or have appetites, or get angry, or feel pity, and in general have pleasure or pain, both too much and too little, and in both ways not well. But having these feelings at the right times, about the right things, toward the right people, for the right end, and in the right way, is the intermediate and best condition, and this is proper to virtue. Similarly, actions also admit of excess, deficiency, and an intermediate condition. (Aristotle 2000, 1106b17–25)

The actor, therefore, is one of the contextual factors that mediates what counts as the mean in a given context. For example, it is virtuous to feel anger when you or your loved ones are insulted or injured, but you not only have to find the mean given the context—the timing, the people involved, the background, the causes of insult, and so on—you also have to consider what your own tendencies are. Are you typically quick to anger, or resentful, or easily enraged? Or do you have a tendency to forgive quickly and easily, to avoid conflict, or to take the other's perspective while neglecting your own injury or unjust treatment? Knowing ourselves and our tendencies with respect to each virtue is necessary to consider when finding the mean in a given context so that we can adjust for our weaknesses and build on our strengths. This is the sense in which Aristotle says that the intermediate condition is "relative to us." Thus, although Aristotle's account of flourishing is integrally bound up in species-specific requirements of basic goods such as nourishment, protection from the environment, friendship, justice, and so on, flourishing cannot be said to be independent of cultural and individual differences. In Douglas Rasmussen's terms (1999), it respects diversity without falling into subjectivism.

This claim can be deceptive, though, because Aristotle's idea of diversity nevertheless holds humans to *one* species-specific aim of actualizing our humanness by achieving excellence. In what follows, I argue that Aristotle's essence-bound position (an essentialist one) of human flourishing is mistaken.

3.2.2 What is wrong with an essential definition of function and, thus, flourishing

Arguments that people are oppressed by structural and systematic injustices are vulnerable to criticisms of essentialism. Adapting this argument from Chris Cuomo's work, I will define essentialism as follows:

1. There are no essences (immutable, ahistorical, eternal, universal, and necessary truths) and therefore no truths about mental health or normality or dysfunction that rely on essences.
2. Various oppressions, adverse living conditions, privileges, and ontological assumptions that affect people who live with distress are created,

enacted, and enforced through definitions of function, flourishing, rationality, and madness that situate many people as Others, both socially and psychologically.

3. Psychiatric theories and practices based on notions that there exist essential features of function/dysfunction, mental health/mental illness, and so on, perpetuate attitudes and values that reduce, mold, and devalue subjects who are afflicted by oppressions and adverse living conditions.

Therefore,

4. Statements such as "People with schizophrenia are unable to make rational decisions to defy psychiatric treatments" attribute essential characteristics to people categorized in that group. Hence, they perpetuate evaluations of people living with distress—or, living very different lives than are believed to lead to flourishing—that are falsely universalizing and, as such, falsely applied to some individual persons. (Adapted from Cuomo 1998, 114.)

Before continuing, I hasten to add that, although I discuss what is mistaken about a philosophical and psychiatric ontology of essences, I do not eschew the reality of material bodies. In particular, it is important for readers to understand that a denial of essentialism need not be a denial of biological human life. Instead, the position is that the biological self is always and unavoidably mediated by beliefs, values, and representations such that the materiality of the body is necessarily embedded and interpreted as a social, moral, political, economic, and biological being. It also is important, when criticizing Aristotle's theory of function and essence, to attend to the dualisms assumed as ontologically natural. Especially problematic are the binaries of functional/dysfunctional, normal/pathological, rational/irrational, and mental illness/mental health. My work challenges these binaries without denying that we are material beings. As Cuomo suggests, we need to "map the contingent, contextually-embedded" ideas of essential nature and function and ensure that we interweave the ways that cultural constructions, practices, and biological matter are formed and reformed (Cuomo 1998, 115). In thinking about Henry's case and others, it is important to steer clear of false universals and, instead, understand that, although metaphysical or ontological truths about function and dysfunction do not exist (particularly in psychiatry), those ontological commitments nevertheless carry immense discursive and physical power (Cuomo 1998, 117). "Discourses motivate, describe, fuel, transform, and limit action in the world" (Cuomo 1998, 124)—that is, we can reject the idea of "Entities with Essences" while acknowledging that "there are real social and ecological beings subsumed under the categories" (Cuomo 1998, 123).

For example, in Henry's case, Cuomo's theory might better capture this particular person as an individual in his own right who is also embedded in cultural and social concepts and practices than would an essentialist account of dysfunction in people with schizophrenia. This embeddedness means that Henry may be evaluated—and may be reflexively embodying—universal ideas about dysfunction in people with schizophrenia. I suggest that such evaluating by psychiatrists and embodying by patients does not entail that universal ideas of dysfunction in patients with schizophrenia are correct. A contextual understanding of his behaviors might resist the assumption that he is dysfunctional in *all* of his defiant behaviors, even though by psychiatric, social, and familial standards he seems to be judged as globally dysfunctional (bracketing off, for the moment, those behaviors that nearly result in his death). Cuomo uses the idea of "dynamic charm," by which she means a being's

> diffuse, "internal" ability to adapt to or resist change, and its unique causal and motivational patterns of behavior—that renders it morally considerable, [roughly, able to be considered as a morally relevant entity] and that serves as a primary site for determining what is good for that being or thing. (Cuomo 1998, 71)

It might be that Henry's dynamic charm is working toward adapting to what is only prima facie "bad" for him and that his resistance to changes such as forced medications and hospitalizations is a positive adaptation of his desire to be morally considerable. I come back to this idea in Chapter 5, adding several caveats.

Cuomo argues that aiming for flourishing involves a conception of the good that is *naturalistic*, meaning grounded in "facts about people, societies, animals, and ecosystemic processes—but that should not be *teleological*—based on the assumption that there exists a determinate final end to which things and processes inevitably aim" (Cuomo 1998, 63; emphasis in original). Cuomo sets out a non-economic and non-instrumental way of valuing. Importantly, such valuing does not require deliberative, rational thought: "In some instances, rational reasons elude us, and we simply *find* ourselves something or some thing that in no meaningful sense can be said to have use value for us" (Cuomo 1998, 64; emphasis in original). Much more needs to be said about rational reasoning as it applies to defiance, and in Section 3.2.3 I begin to develop this crucial topic.

3.2.3 Aristotle's account of flourishing as excellent reasoning

Although I discuss reasoning and epistemology in more depth in Chapters 5 and 6, here I identify problems with Aristotle's integral connection between flourishing and his conception of reasoning. Aristotle makes a tight connection between having character virtue and having the virtue of *phronesis*. *Phronesis* is both a necessary and sufficient virtue because one cannot fully have the virtues of character and fail to exercise this central virtue of thought. *Phronesis* involves good deliberation about what promotes good ends, being able to grasp particulars while understanding the relevant universals, and then making correct inferences from universal principles to action and consciousness (Aristotle 1985, 1142bff; see Dahl 1984 for a complete analysis of Aristotle's *phronesis*).

This is a demanding requirement for flourishing and *eudaimonia*, and its legacy is still prevalent in normative conceptions of rationality—norms that are embedded in psychiatry and that shape diagnosis and treatment. But behavior can still be spontaneous if we create the background conditions for good decision-making. Iris Murdoch discusses this point in *The sovereignty of good*: "I can only choose within the world I can *see*, in the moral sense of "see" which implies that clear vision is a result of moral imagination and moral effort" (Murdoch 1970, 37; emphasis in original). A background of good moral vision and just relations is compatible with the need for defiant acts to be "sense-making" even when those acts are not, in the moment, deliberated about in the unfolding of defiance. So defiance is made intelligible not necessarily by evident in-the-moment *phronesis*, but by the defier's ability to give post hoc "reasonableness" explanations of defiance's expression. These explanations may be based on background deliberation, or they may draw upon tacit knowing. My definition of tacit knowing is a combination of intuition and inference, where the process in coming to know can be constructed post hoc (unlike intuitive knowing, which remains inchoate). For example, a clinician may intuit some of the signs that a patient is giving, such as that the patient is angry with her clinician; the clinician both draws on her gut feelings and "picks up" the way the patient is presenting at the moment. This can also be the case for a patient. Henry, let's say, may draw on tacit reasoning when he escapes hospitals and refuses to take his medications. He may be able to offer post hoc reasons—for example, that he has magical experiences that he does not want to suppress just because others think he is sick. His reasons are likely to be interpreted as falling outside norms of rationality, but then we must interrogate norms of rationality and not merely acquiesce to their power. I return to this point shortly.

The second point about the place of reasoning in flourishing is that critical reflection may be especially important for those whose characters have become normalized as submissive and compliant. Tessman suggests that, upon reflection, many oppressed people come to regret the self that they have become and that agent-regret, coupled with anger, is a necessary step toward creating liberatory feminist virtues (2005, 12–13). Learning to be defiant, then, will involve practicing new responses that, in turn, will require learning to identify situations that call for defiance rather than acquiescence or civility—but that are not excessive. The point is that those living under adverse conditions, especially those with mental disabilities, need to develop a kind of practical reason. I develop this point in Chapter 5.

The third problem of the relationship of reasoning to defiant actions concerns the nature of reasoning itself. As I argue elsewhere, norms of rationality are, in part, political, because they not only frame the parameters for acceptable behavior, they also set a standard for socially permissible desires (Potter 2002). If Henry, for example, reflected and was willing to take the risk that swimming naked in freezing water might end his life, his desire would be counted as suicidal, and suicide is normatively irrational. The prescriptiveness of dominant rationality constrains not only behavior and desires, but also discourse itself.

> The problem is that the norms for rationality have been established by a politically powerful public who have excluded certain people from having a voice in either criticizing or expanding the norms. When marginalized groups attempt to offer arguments as to why the norms need to be expanded, the arguments are judged according to the very standards of rationality they are trying to challenge, and unless their criticisms stay within accepted boundaries, their arguments will likely be rejected as irrational. As a result, these groups stay excluded from the discourse, while the norms remain secure. (Potter 2002, 49–50)

This point is applicable especially to those with mental distress and disabilities, who may struggle with having their voice given uptake and being understood on their own terms. It also applies to those whose behavior is interpreted—not necessarily correctly—as mental dysfunction, examples of which I discuss in Chapter 4. In this chapter, Henry is one example of such a struggle, and the case of Rachel, discussed in Section 3.3, is another.

Fourth, a deep concern I have with emphasizing *phronesis* in the development of defiance is that defiance itself can be disciplined. Aristotle is clear that, in practical reason, intellect leads to decision-making and the passions must be corralled and reined in. This governing of passion by intellect assures that the right ratio of rationality to appetite is found. Unruly appetites, or those that threaten to dominate practical reason and mislead us, must be suppressed. The problem is that we need some degree of *phronesis* in order to get it right with defiance and other virtues, but *phronesis* by its very nature is disciplining and taming—meaning that it disciplines and tames the passions. By this I mean that any move toward striking the Aristotelian mean is a socializing move. So, to exhibit the virtue, we must necessarily also shift the weight from its characteristics proper to a domesticated and less-frightening-to-others approach. The more we tether defiance to reason, the less likely we are to be able to retain two of the characteristics that can be valuable about defiance—its unboundedness and its passion.

So, I worry that defiance tamed would be a loss for the disenfranchised. Still, I suggest that critical reflection about oppressive norms and structures is necessary to liberatory praxis—even though it is not helpful in the moment of spontaneous defiance. Among other things, we could reflect on the effectiveness and objectives of defiant acts. There is a place for critical reflection: for defiance to be genuinely empowering and efficacious, it most likely has to be taken up and reflected upon at a collective level. By this I mean that the benefits of defiance might include an assertion of self-respect or a communication of one's moral worth. But holding oneself as a self-respecting being in the face of oppressive power structures does not reach very far into the future in bringing about sociopolitical and economic change. Individual acts of defiance, therefore, may not be particularly empowering or liberating. That is, they may be empowering for the individual in the moment, but they are not strengthened by connection with a wider community. For more on this, see my contrast between defiance and civil disobedience in Chapter 2. Also, because defiance is a virtue, it has an excess, and a consistently defiant person has a vice. I do not assume or equate that having a vice of defiance indicates a mental disorder, however. What the parameters of good defiance are and how and why defiance can be a bad thing are taken up in Chapter 5, beginning with a case of someone who might be diagnosed with Antisocial Personality Disorder.

Finally, Chapter 2 identified a problem with being defiant, namely that the consequences may be very costly; I return to this issue at the end of Chapter 4. This problem harks back to Tessman's argument that flourishing may not be possible in the world we live in, where multiple oppressions, disabilities, and mental disorders abound. One of the reasons that flourishing is unreachable is that the very actions that would move struggling people toward a more flourishing life are ones that are impeded, constrained, and, in many cases, severely punished. Tessman does not think that eudaimonism should be jettisoned altogether, and I agree: we need a conception of non-ideal flourishing that provides a picture for people who are variously oppressed and disabled to strive for liberation.

But what would a conception of non-ideal flourishing be like, in particular for those with mental disabilities?

3.3 **Flourishing and mental disorder**

In this section, I focus on the relationship between flourishing and mental disorder. For many clinicians, patients, and family members of patients, it is hard to imagine the possibility of living a flourishing life under mental distress, problems in work and relationships, and, often, accompanying physical problems. This discussion begins to construct a realistic but hopeful view of just some of the components of flourishing under duress. I start with a literature review that suggests to me that, in attempting to shift from the mental illness traits in the mental illness/mental health binary to that of mental health, a conception of flourishing is unrealistic and discouraging—at least as it is being conceived there.

3.3.1 **Current work from psychiatry and psychology on flourishing**

The movement called positive psychology holds that it is past time we paid attention to mental health so that policies and practices can understand what it is and how to promote it (Huppert and So 2013; Chida and Steptoe 2008; Deiner, Helliwell, and Kahneman 2010; Dolan, Peasgood, and White 2008; Huppert 2009; Lyubomirsky, King, and Diener 2005). The idea is that positive emotions, attitudes, and states can promote mental health, and that focusing exclusively on treating mental illness and preventing it is insufficient to foster well-being in people (see Box 3.1). As Corey Keyes puts it, the focus on reducing and preventing mental illnesses

> rests on one of the most simple and inexplicably untested empirical hypotheses: The absence of mental illness is the presence of mental health. Put in psychometric terminology, the success of the current approach to mental health hinges on the hypothesis that measures of mental illness and measures of mental health belong to a single, bipolar latent continuum. (Keyes 2007, 95)

Keyes, and many others, hold that "the absence of mental illness is not the presence of mental health" (2007, 95). Clearly, a debate exists regarding how to conceptualize the relationship of mental health to mental illness. Keyes and some others argue for a two-continua model, whereas Hubbard and So and others place mental health and illness on opposite ends of one continuum (Keyes 2007; Hubbard and So 2013). Among the many approaches, the common thread is the view that well-being is multi-dimensional (Hubbard and So 2013).

It is important to note that, in the literature, well-being is interpreted as flourishing. Huppert and So (2013) define flourishing as "the experience of life going well," "a combination of feeling good and functioning effectively"

Box 3.1 Positive psychology

In the late twentieth century, a movement began called "positive psychology." Critics of typical foci of psychology became concerned with the emphasis in research and therapeutic treatments of the field on how people can learn to cope with stress, grief, disease, and dysfunctional lives. They began promoting values of what constitutes a meaningful life in psychology and for patients. Positive psychology helps patients orient themselves toward attitudes of engagement with others and in the world, instead of a narrower focus in therapy on the individual's problems and stressors. Although proponents of this view agree that patients need assistance in coping with crises and with problems in living, and that additional research on this topic is still needed, they also think that too much attention to negative aspects of living is inadequate in helping the patient in the long run. Values in positive psychology include creativity, optimism, beneficence toward others, and identification of what would make a meaningful life for patients. The theory that underlies positive psychology is one of flourishing, where flourishing requires that one lives a life of virtue (see Keyes and Haidt 2003).

"as synonymous with a high level of mental well-being, it epitomizes mental health" (2013, 838). This parallels another distinction in the positive psychology literature, between hedonic well-being (life satisfaction and subjective well-being) and eudaimonistic well-being (more objective human functioning). That is, eudaimonistic well-being is viewed as necessary to overall flourishing because findings show that hedonic well-being alone is insufficient to measure overall well-being (Huppart and So 2013).

Typically, eudemonistic flourishing is tied to human functioning, such as in "developing nascent abilities and capacities toward becoming a more fully functioning person and citizen" (Keyes 2006, 396). I reject such a strong tie with human function, for reasons I gave in Section 3.2.1. But Keyes unpacks his concept of flourishing in other research. In assessing the rate of flourishing among adolescents, Keyes measures social contribution, social integration, social actualization, social acceptance, and social coherence (see Table 3.A for an explanation of Keyes' assessment criteria).

In general, both hedonic and eudaimonistic measures are included in determining the flourishing of groups of people. Positive features of mental health are identified as competence, emotional stability, engagement, meaning,

Table 3.A Measuring subjective well-being in youth

Social contribution	"How often did you feel that you had something important to contribute to society?"
Social integration	"How often did you feel that you belonged to a community like a social group, your school, or your neighborhood?"
Social actualization	"How often did you feel that our society is becoming a better place?"
Social acceptance	"How often did you feel that people are basically good?"
Social coherence	"How often did you feel that the way our society works made sense to you?"

Source: Keyes 2006, 397.

optimism, positive emotion, positive relationships, resilience, self-esteem, and vitality. Table 3.B, used in the European Social Survey (ESS), shows the common values and measures for flourishing: the items on the left are widely considered to be the ten components of flourishing.

Huppert and So's operational definition of flourishing is that "in order to qualify as flourishing, a person had to show the presence of positive emotion together with all but one of the positive characteristics and all but one aspect of positive functioning" (2013, 852). Interestingly, the ESS findings, when analyzing flourishing, reveal cross-cultural difference across European countries: Denmark has the highest rate of flourishing (40.6 percent) while Slovakia, the Russian Federation, and Portugal have the lowest. Huppert and So note that the countries that report people with the highest rate of flourishing are also the ones with relative wealth and low income inequality; "Explanations include well-developed social welfare and health care systems, low unemployment, high social trust, and ethnic homogeneity" (Huppert and So 2013, 852). Low social trust is consistently correlated with low well-being (e.g., Dolan, Peasgood, and White 2008).

Contrary to most evidence, both from positive psychology and from empirical evidence in schools, prisons, ghettoized neighborhoods, and health care treatment, Keyes reports that Black people in America have an advantage in flourishing and that no gender disparity exists in flourishing among whites (Keyes 2009, 2007). Keyes suggests that an advantage is conferred on Black people through racial socialization and group identification. He argues that these characteristics "instill meaning, purpose, pride, and commitment to the goal of self-development" (2009, 1692). He suggests two explanations: that Black parents are more concerned with helping the next generation and so

Table 3.B Features of flourishing and indicator items from the European Social Survey

Positive feature	ESS item used as indicator
Competence	Most days I feel a sense of accomplishment from what I do
Emotional stability	(In the past week) I felt calm and peaceful
Engagement	I love learning new things
Meaning	I generally feel that what I do in my life is valuable and worthwhile
Optimism	I am always optimistic about my future
Positive emotion	Taking all things together, how happy would you say you are?
Positive relationships	There are people in my life who really care about me
Resilience	When things go wrong in my life it generally takes me a long time to get back to normal (reverse score)
Self-esteem	In general, I feel very positive about myself
Vitality	(In the past week) I had a lot of energy

Reproduced by permission from: Felicia Huppert and Timothy So. 2013. Flourishing across Europe: Application of a new conceptual framework for defining well-being, *Social Indicators Research* 110 (3):837–61.

view themselves as role models, and that narrative life stories incorporate themes of contamination and redemption. According to Keyes, both of these strategies for living with inequality contribute to mental resilience and greater well-being.

The evidence I discuss in Chapters 3 and 4 flies in the face of Keyes' claims. Whether we are talking about people whose living conditions are oppressive or people who are living with mental disabilities—and often they go together—resilience, meaning, and sense-making of the current world are strained or damaged for many people. My general assessment of the conception of flourishing found in positive psychology is that it articulates neatly with psychiatric values of function and dysfunction but fails to present realistic norms for flourishing that would speak to and resonate with the mentally struggling and distressed.

A more promising account of flourishing for people with mental illnesses can be found in the work of Martha Nussbaum. Nussbaum presents a theory of basic powers or capabilities that people are able to perform (2006). (See Box 3.2 for information on Nussbaum's list of basic capabilities.) The idea of basic capabilities was first articulated by Amartya Sen, whose ideas emerged from his work on economics and development in poor countries and among poor people (Sen 1985). Nussbaum (2006) argues that a just society will organize

Box 3.2 An outline of Nussbaum's list of ten basic capabilities

1. Life. Being able to live to the end of a human life of normal length; not dying prematurely.
2. Bodily health. Being able to have good health, including reproductive health; being adequately nourished; being able to have adequate shelter.
3. Bodily integrity. Being able to move freely from place to place; being able to be secure against violent assault, including sexual assault; having opportunities for sexual satisfaction and for choice in matters of reproduction.
4. Senses, imagination, thought. Being able to use the senses; being able to imagine, to think, and to reason—and to do these things in a way informed and cultivated by an adequate education; being able to use imagination and thought in connection with experiencing, and producing expressive works and events of one's own choice; being able to use one's mind in ways protected by guarantees of freedom of expression with respect to both political and artistic speech and freedom of religious exercise; being able to have pleasurable experiences and to avoid nonbeneficial pain.
5. Emotions. Being able to have attachments to things and persons outside ourselves; being able to love those who love and care for us; being able to grieve at their absence, to experience longing, gratitude, and justified anger; not having one's emotional developing blighted by fear or anxiety.
6. Practical reason. Being able to form a conception of the good and to engage in critical reflection about the planning of one's own life. (This entails protection for liberty of conscience.)
7. Affiliation. Being able to live for and in relation to others, to recognize and show concern for other human beings, to engage in various forms of social interaction; being able to imagine the situation of another and to have compassion for that situation; having the capability for both justice and friendship. Being able to be treated as a dignified being whose worth is equal to that of others.
8. Other species. Being able to live with concern for and in relation to animals, plants, and the world of nature.
9. Play. Being able to laugh, to play, to enjoy recreational activities.

10. Control over one's environment. Includes both political control: being able to participate effectively in political choices that govern one's life; having the rights of political participation, free speech and freedom of association; and material control: being able to hold property (both land and movable goods); having the right to seek employment on an equal basis with others. (Nussbaum 2006, 76–8)

policy, institutions, and education such that people with mental disabilities have access to basic capabilities.

Nussbaum's account of capabilities provides an idea of what makes living well possible, while at the same time it does not assume that people will want to explore or develop those capabilities. That is, she distinguishes between having these capabilities and exercising them. One might choose not to exercise a capability, but it is a violation of a human right to prevent one from developing these capabilities. A just society will provide support for capabilities of those who live with mental disabilities. Lack of proper care, or inadequate care, that otherwise would lend support for basic capabilities to be realized are indicators of an unjust society. The relevance of Nussbaum's work to mentally ill patients who are defiant is found in the connection between capabilities and mental disabilities. As I understand Nussbaum's argument, support for capabilities for people living with mental disabilities does not entail flourishing but provides the conditions that would make flourishing possible. Impediments to the development and expression of capabilities may, then, give the individual reasons to be defiant. If one's ability to access or express basic powers inherent in human life is structurally blocked or immobilized, or is unsupported through adequate resources and good psychiatric care, then defiance may be the appropriate response.

Still, I am hesitant to endorse the capabilities approach wholeheartedly. My primary reservation is that Nussbaum's argument for the existence of essential and basic powers is not far from Aristotle's claims about the essence of human function. Indeed, Nussbaum is unapologetically an Aristotelian essentialist (see Nussbaum 1992). While I do ascribe to the existence of the material human body, with its basic needs and demands, I believe that the material body is always mediated by culture and society. In addition, any tight connection between essential human needs or capabilities (or virtues) and rationality ought to be met with skepticism and resistance, as I argued in Section 3.2.2.

3.4 **Some components of non-ideal flourishing**

So what is flourishing, then, according to my analysis? Let me begin by returning to Tessman's work on burdened virtues and reminding ourselves of what the absence of flourishing involves. In discussing a domain of virtue neglected by Aristotle, Tessman suggests that suffering is a result of human action and therefore is potentially preventable. Examples she gives are of poverty, child abuse, violence against women, political torture, slavery, and genocide. Suffering is great, and unjust, but it is ignorable; people can remain indifferent to it, or willfully ignorant of it. Yet, Tessman says, "The background conditions of the world we live in make it impossible to escape both the horror of indifference and the psychic pain (and perhaps exhaustion) of sensitivity and attention" (Tessman 2005).

Following Tessman's lead, I suggest that what we should be looking for is a modest set of traits that serve to benefit and, potentially, liberate people to some degree. I quote Tessman extensively here because her voice says it best. The idea I track is that some virtue traits serve as important guides for living even though those traits need not give the promise that they lead to flourishing:

> Failing to connect (straightforwardly) to a good life need not disqualify a trait from being a virtue, precisely because virtue is insufficient for flourishing; under adverse conditions, traits that still can be assessed as virtues may fail to manifest any connection to a good life. These are the burdened virtues. (Tessman 2005)

For example, a burdened virtue might be feeling too much anguish at the suffering of others, such that the self is neglected or unable to thrive. I have suggested also that a burdened virtue might be acquiescent behavior in the face of authority—including psychiatric authority—when one might feel more self-worth by being defiant. But a burdened virtue might also be one where being defiant as a psychiatric patient benefits one in terms of confirming self-worth or integrity but still damages the self through consequences from others (such as forced medications or involuntary hospitalization).

Tessman makes a useful distinction here between trait guidance (guidance in what is a choiceworthy trait, or is best to choose, in a given situation) and trait assessment (the assessment of that trait as a good one, i.e., as a virtue). This distinction calls attention to the way that what counts as a choiceworthy trait given the circumstances is not the same as saying that it is a good or virtuous trait. Tessman's point is that, under oppressive or disadvantaged circumstances, trait guidance and trait assessment can come apart. She argues that, in some cases where trait guidance and trait assessment come apart, an action may not be a virtue, but that in other cases, it may be. This is because being virtuous is frequently disconnected from flourishing. We can see this better by considering different types of traits that might count as virtues.

In trait v_1, guidance and assessment go together:

> Trait v_1 tends to enable its bearer to make the right decisions and to perform good actions (given the assumption that these are available); and, having trait v_1 is conducive to or partly constitutes living a good life. (Tessman 2005)

Bearers of trait v_1, then, are dispositionally situated to express a virtue. I will argue that some defiant behavior fits trait v_1. However, sometimes what is best to choose in a given circumstance occasions regret or heartache. When good actions are available but are accompanied by moral residue, they might better fit trait v_2:

> Trait v_2 tends to enable its bearer to choose as well as possible, with the appropriate feelings, such as regret or anguish, toward what cannot be done. Furthermore, trait v_2 is a trait that would be good—in the straightforward sense of conducive to or constitutive of flourishing—if conditions were better and presented a truly good option, for in such a case v_2 would operate without the encumbrance of a moral remainder, and thus without the negative feelings that attach to it. (Tessman 2005)

As Tessman explains, and as Chapter 2 suggests, trait guidance and trait assessment frequently come apart, especially for those living under adverse conditions. Trait v_2 thus characterizes a burdened virtue. Yet it is a good course to choose, and it would be good in an uncompromised sense if circumstances were such that it was not accompanied by moral regret or distress. Sometimes, however, even this degree of link between trait guidance and trait assessment is not available:

> Trait v_3 is chosen because it is judged to be the best trait to cultivate in the circumstances, even though it is not conducive to or constitutive of anyone's flourishing at present; it does, however, tend to enable its bearer to perform actions with the aim of eventually making flourishing lives more possible overall (for the bearer of trait v_3 and/or for others). (Tessman 2005)

Trait v_3 is good to develop for future, but not current, flourishing. The case of Büschler from Chapter 2 might be an example of trait v_3 defiance in her circumstances. Büschler may have developed a disposition to be defiant that primarily or solely benefits other women in the future. Some defiant patients may be expressing virtue as found in trait v_1, while others may express defiance as a virtue in the sense of traits v_2 or v_3. That is, while some defiance may be burdened, it is not always a burdened virtue. This point is explicated in Chapter 4, where I conclude with reasons why defiance is, sometimes, choice-worthy *and* good. However, Chapter 4 also gives reasons why defiance might sometimes better fit the following type of trait:

> Trait v_4 tends to enable its bearer to make the best possible decisions and to perform the best possible actions; and, having trait v_4 is conducive to or partly constitutes living as well as possible, though because trait v_4 carries a cost to its bearer (and perhaps to others), it is only choiceworthy when bad conditions are present and a good life is unattainable. (Tessman 2005)

For some people, trait v_4 may be the best they can hope for. I do not think that defiance can only fall under a trait v_4 kind (although it sometimes will do so). Even when it does, however, Tessman is careful to caution against despair. A focus on this trait allows us to keep *eudaimonia* in sight while eschewing hopelessness:

> The choice to go on living, to insist upon life—with its sufferings and its joys—is an existential choice of great significance under oppression, and this choice captures something crucial about eudaimonism. In fact, this phenomenon of affirming life may offer insights into how one is to conceive of any human flourishing, for in choosing life one chooses what is at the core of a good life. (Tessman 2005)

From this framework, I am able to articulate some features of flourishing worth aiming at that do not require an ontological commitment to human functioning or Aristotelian essentialism or a rosy view of mental health. Flourishing, then, would seem to include at least the following elements:

(1) giving and receiving attentiveness, sensitivity, and positive concern for great suffering without destroying the self;
(2) an adequate recognition of interdependence that entails mutuality;
(3) a reduction in moral damage;
(4) a decrease in the existence of burdened virtues;
(5) access to the expression of basic capabilities.

I include (5) only if the essential human qualities entailed in capabilities are not attached to, or ontologically committed to, the idea that a being's function identifies its essence and that, for humans, that essence is rationality (see Section 3.2.1). These features of flourishing set a realistic and hopeful standard that can guide particular virtue traits in people. Nevertheless, as I argued in Chapter 2, it is important to remember that some people who live with severe mental illness, with or without the added constraints of structurally disadvantaged living conditions, may be unable to experience any of those qualities of flourishing. For some people, or in some situations, flourishing simply may not be possible. Additionally, note that that the features of non-ideal flourishing I set out do not indicate a specific line between flourishing and living without any degree of flourishing at all. With that framework for non-ideal flourishing in place, I turn to two more cases to see how the discussion of this chapter might be applied.

3.5 **Depression and defiance**

Depression, generalized anxiety disorder, and mixed depression and anxiety have the highest prevalence of all mental illnesses in the European and U.S. populations (Huppert and So 2013). Depression is projected to become even more prevalent worldwide (Murray and Lopez 1996). It has the potential to be one of the most debilitating and disabling of illnesses (see Solomon 2002). In some cases, it is difficult to imagine that clinical therapy that focuses on working toward flourishing by cultivating liberatory virtues would be very helpful. Yet it might be.

3.5.1 **Marie**

Marie is utterly defeated. She suffers from severe depression. She grew up wanting to be a nurse. Her father abused her, and her mother scared her; Marie describes her mother as "a witch." Talking about the past does not relieve her pain. Anti-depressants are prescribed, changed, and changed again when they too fail to offer relief. She occasionally self-medicates with heroin. She has a remission, during which time she learns how to mend computer hardware, only for her depression to descend upon her again. Lauren Slater, her clinician, describes Marie as numb and paralyzed by her depression:

> She had just woken up that morning and felt the dread of that depression back on her. She had tried to get out of bed and found she could barely move. The idea of facing what just yesterday she had loved appalled her. The wires would look ugly, rotting tendons on greased machines. The gas plasma screens would reek, glow a fetid green. She couldn't go. She just couldn't go. Her heart hammered and every second squeezed inside. Morning passed into noon, noon into dusk. (Slater 1996, 127)

Marie takes an accidental overdose of heroin and ends up in the hospital. In the psychiatric unit, Marie refuses to come out of her room except to spend hours in the toilet; she weeps for hours, and she is adamant about not attending groups.

Surprisingly, her therapist Lauren Slater says about this refusal:

> I was actually happy to hear about Marie's refusal to go to groups. It spoke of some spark of anger, some spot still scarlet within her. When I heard that, I got yet another glimpse of Marie, this time not joyful, not flattened by grief, but lit red in her rage. (Slater 1996, 129)

I suggest that Marie is guided by a nascent virtue—perhaps one that maps onto Tessman's trait v_3. Although embryonic, it has the potential to develop into a virtue that can guide her through and out of some of the darkness, paralysis, and despair that have held her captive. That virtue is defiance.

Slater has homed in on a key issue in defiance: that what prima facie is a right to refuse treatment may, because of the passion behind refusal, be more like a defiant act. Slater uses language such as "spark of anger" and "lit red in her rage" to characterize Marie's new state, one that gives Slater a glimpse of what Marie can become. Marie is not merely refusing to go to groups from a well-reasoned position where she has weighed various pros and cons and decided to make a decision not to go to group. Instead, she has tapped into anger about her depression and the seeming hopelessness of her condition. That anger breathes life into her in a way that rejects a despondent, numb self. In refusing to go to groups out of anger and rage, Marie engages her own stronger self. And a central part of expressing that angry self is that she moves toward defying norms of the patient role, of depressed women as dependent and helpless, and even the norm that psychiatric hospitals can begin to heal patients through socializing them. The distinction between the right to refuse treatment and the expression of defiant acts is blurred here, but the markers that Marie is exhibiting defiance are her passionate engagement with her own stronger self—something that was itself depressed for most of her life.

In reflecting on how a norm of flourishing would function in Marie's case, I believe that an act of defiance—even an apparently minor one such as refusing to attend group activities—moves her, ever so slightly, toward liberation from her depression. The features of flourishing I have in mind are (3), (4), and (5) from Section 3.4: a decrease in a burdened virtue, a reduction in moral damage, and access to capabilities. The claim that Marie's defiance is a decrease in a burdened virtue needs to be explained. Marie is aware of norms for compliant patient behavior and has tried to follow those norms in her treatment with Slater. The hospital also has expectations of and norms for its patients. In both situations, those norms typically are reasonable ones, and the psychiatrists and therapists who work with Marie and other patients are aiming at the good in endorsing those norms. Yet in Marie's case, where severe depression interacts with those norms of compliance, Marie experiences herself as confined, immobilized, and trapped, and she becomes subservient in order to suppress those bad feelings. The subservience and acquiescence she sometimes exhibits is a burdened virtue, in the sense of Tessman's trait v_4. Now, it is true that we are not always the best judge of what is good for us and that we objectively can be wrong about being subjugated. In some cases, defiance would not be considered good. But, from my understanding of Marie's story, I think she is objectively subjugated through her childhood and subsequent depression and thus lives with burdened virtues. Trait v_4 burdened virtues do not serve Marie well—they do not contribute to her flourishing and, indeed, seem to impede it—and so Marie finally gets angry while in hospital. I would argue that her defiance, in the form of anger, shifts her from a trait v_4 burdened virtue to trait v_2 or even to trait v_1. I am not sure whether or not anger is partly constitutive of a good life, but I am inclined to think that it is. In an ideal world, where flourishing is possible for all (or nearly all), would reasonable anger still have a place? I think so. Removing structural barriers to economic parity, social equality, and adequate material resources would not eliminate the possibility that someone might be insulting or hurtful to oneself or one's loved ones, and in such situations anger would be the appropriate response. As Aristotle says, a "willingness to accept insults to oneself and to overlook insults to one's family and friends is slavish" (1999, NE 1126a10). I would allow for the explanation that her anger might itself be burdened, but I believe that, at the least, it expresses a *lighter* burden. Defiance, in Marie's case, taps into one of Nussbaum's capabilities. The capability I have in mind is Nussbaum's number five regarding emotions, which specifically states that one of the emotions is justified anger, where experiencing anger is a basic good (Nussbaum 2000, 77; see also Nussbaum 2003). I can imagine that Marie's defiant behavior allows her to experience a basic power, and that experience is strengthening and life-affirming. It is objectively better than being submissive and crushed by circumstances and mental illness. By refusing to comply with staff expectations and by asserting herself as someone who will not submit to something she does not like and does not believe will help her, Marie shifts away from moral damage. And perhaps, within Marie, such an act of defiance decreases her relationship to burdened virtues: by refusing, with passion and energy, to attend group activities, she reorients herself toward what she can do and not what she cannot do; she chooses within constraints, but decides what she wants for herself despite the authoritative structure of the hospital (allowing that, in many other cases, the authority of psychiatrists is in the direction of what is good for the patient) and she chooses without a negative remainder of feeling. Her anger and passion see her through this.

Marie's therapist plays an important role in Marie's shift toward these features of flourishing. Slater affirms and reinforces Marie's defiance. There are two ways that liberatory defiance is not strictly individualistic: one is that it requires uptake from another, a reminder of our relationality; another is that, although sometimes defiant acts are concerned with the particular individual and are self-interested—not focused on whether or how defiance might benefit others—defiance and other virtues that benefit the oppressed, the disadvantaged, and the disabled are best thought of as encompassing concern for others' liberation as well as one's own. This second point is more difficult to act on for psychiatric patients because, so often, they are both psychically and socially isolated from others and a passionate conception of defiance cannot extend beyond what is good for them. This is one reason why giving uptake to defiance is so important. I explain the virtue of giving uptake in Chapter 6.

3.6 **Borderline personality disorder**

The "borderline" patient represents the quintessential noncompliant patient (see Potter 2009). Borderline Personality Disorder (BPD) is characterized by identity disturbance, feelings of chronic emptiness, impulsive or self-destructive behavior, and unstable intense interpersonal relationships. Emotional dysregulation, cognitive distortions such as all-or nothing thinking, and splitting others into a good/bad dichotomy are also central. This last section presents the case of Rachel, a case that is challenging for its complexity in understanding flourishing and defiance.

Rachel had been seeing her psychiatrist for some time when she first received her diagnosis of BPD. She came into his office, infuriated:

> "Bullshit! This is all bullshit. I signed so much crap in the hospital, filled out so many forms. Who reads it all anyway? A bunch of bureaucratic, psychobabble paperwork bullshit. You're a chickenshit; that's what you are, a spineless chicken shit. From that very first session when you didn't have the balls to give me the test results to my face, just tossed me some goddamn written report on my way out the door. And now I've got some psycho, demented mental illness. I despise you. I wish I had never ever met you."
>
> By now the drum roll had reached peak intensity, the chair not only swiveling, but rocking back and forth, my feet tapping the floor, body shaking, ready to explode.
>
> "Rachel, you're an adult. You're not crazy, and you can control your body motion. Stop with the tapping, stop with the feet and the chair, calm down, and listen."
>
> Without raising his voice in the slightest, he had delivered his command with clear authority. Still seething, I stopped moving.
>
> "First of all, you know the rules here. We can't work on your intense feelings when you physically act them out. We need to use words."
>
> "Okay then. Fuck you." (Reiland 2004, 123)

Rachel is justifiably pissed off: a crucial aspect of her treatment—her diagnosis—has been kept from her. She wonders why. Is it because her psychiatrist does not think she can handle the information? Is it because the diagnosis is so devastating? Rachel experiences the *suppression* of her diagnosis to be devastating, a betrayal of trust between her psychiatrist and her. She is abusive, which alienates her from the primary person who can be her ally. She acts out, which is unproductive in liberating her from the burdened virtue of submission. But when she uses words to express her fury, she is closer to the mean of defiance. She takes a huge, somewhat calculated risk in letting her psychiatrist know how painful and infuriating this is. Because she is doing what he asks, she catches him in the irony of the authority of words.

I like the feistiness of Rachel's response and think it merits consideration as a contender for "good" defiance. While her defiance is mixed, it moves her closer to a more liberating way of refusing submission to her psychiatrist's action of withholding her diagnosis while maintaining her relationship with him. She is experimenting with shedding a burdened (trait v_4) virtue—that of submissiveness—while at the same time trying on a form of defiance that is, to some degree, more constructively communicative than what she had previously been doing. She begins to shed some of her most abusive tactics that come out of moral damage. Defiance, for Rachel, is not yet dispositionally good, but it is behavior that, if practiced well, can eventually become a virtue at least in Tessman's trait v_2 sense. It might even be that Rachel's defiance, if developed properly, would fall under the category of trait v_1 for choiceworthy action. Having the virtue of defiance, as I have articulated it, is a readiness to be defiant when situations call for it. Although the locus of concern in my book is on defiance as a virtue for the disadvantaged or the oppressed, I do not think that the need for defiant behavior is tied only to circumstances that are unjustly constraining. In other words, defiance may sometimes be an unburdened virtue, and I am suggesting that Rachel's defiance may eventually become an unburdened virtue. This is not the same as claiming that Rachel eventually will live a flourishing life, but only to say that defiance is partly constitutive of such a life.

While Rachel herself does not frame issues this way, I suggest a socially contextual interpretation that helps situate her behavior and my claims about her better defiance. Rachel is likely to be beset with gender stereotypes that hinder her development and striving for any semblance of flourishing. Her defiance of her psychiatrist's authority allows her to flaunt conversational norms that govern the therapeutic relationship. Rachel may need this defiance in order to heal from damage wrought by a hegemonic and sexist society. Furthermore, BPD is itself gender-biased, both in its criteria for diagnosis and in its conception and treatment of its largely female patient population (Potter 2009). Rachel arguably has reasons besides an individualist dysfunctional explanation for her behavior toward her psychiatrist. It may be true that her defiant and abusive behavior stems from emotional dysregulation, a problem that many people with BPD encounter. That is, multiple causes may exist for her defiant behavior. The point I am making is that, even in the context of a personality disorder (if she has one, which Rachel herself comes to accept [Reiland 2004]), her defiance may be a reasonable response aimed at flourishing. Her status as gendered has intersected with her learning of her diagnosis and her confrontation of her psychiatrist to position her as defiant—an assessment that, to her psychiatrist, may signify emotional dysregulation, but that could simultaneously signify appropriate defiance in the sociohistorical context of her life.

Rachel's case differs from the previous cases in this chapter (Henry and Marie), in that I set the analysis of Rachel's defiance in the context of broader social concerns, namely continuing gender stereotypes, inequalities, and persistent sexism. But each of these cases exemplifies struggles with the relationship between mental illness and flourishing and, in Henry's case, the oppressive potential of psychiatry. In each of these cases, I take seriously Tessman's argument that a theory of non-ideal flourishing is important to retain. I revisit the question of whether or not Henry's defiance contributes to his flourishing in Chapter 5 when I analyze the difference between good and bad defiance. Chapter 4 delves more deeply into questions of burdened virtues, risks, and flourishing through an examination of defiant behavior in children.

Chapter 4

Interpreting defiant behavior in children: Constructs, norms, and intersectionalities

In this chapter, I analyze current research on aggression. The focus is on children's aggressive behavior that sometimes yields a diagnosis of Oppositional Defiant Disorder (ODD). I argue that the distinctions drawn in types of aggression do not yield a construct or model that is clear. I suggest that the norms that determine harms and violations worth meriting the characterization of aggressive behavior need to be articulated and critiqued. Additionally, I complicate the often simplistic distinctions drawn between genders in these discussions by examining the matrix of raced, gendered, and classed intersections in the interpretation and reproduction of norms for behavior. By taking up these issues, I call attention to the challenges that many teachers and clinicians face when interpreting children's behavior as defiant, aggressive, and worthy of interventions.

The progression of my argument is as follows. In Section 4.2, I set out the characteristics of ODD and Conduct Disorder (CD) in order to prepare for a discussion and analysis of the larger context for understanding defiant behavior. Section 4.3 explains why I think that the construct of aggression is flawed. In Sections 4.4 and 4.5 I present features of aggression in children's play and then analyze children's play in terms of their hegemonic struggles. I will then be in a position to analyze defiant behavior using the concept of intersectionalities in Section 4.6, where I argue that defiance may be misread and misinterpreted if the knowledge and tools from this analysis are not employed. At the end of the chapter, I consider the reasons children (and adults) might have for being defiant of some of the prevailing norms, even at risk of retribution or clinical intervention. The aims of the chapter are twofold: first, I want to make clear to psychiatrists and teachers how a deeper analysis of the construct of aggression makes it much more difficult to interpret certain behavior as maladaptive defiant traits; and, second, I hope to encourage a more deliberative and critical process in interpreting such behavior.

I begin with the work of ethnographer Ruth Woods (2013), who studied children's moral development at a large multicultural school in West London. One of the children in her study was Paul, whose escalating physical aggression raises the question, in my mind, of whether or not Paul might be heading toward the development of ODD or a future diagnosis of CD—in other words, whether his aggression should be considered a kind of "bad" defiance. A discussion of Paul's case is threaded throughout this chapter and Chapter 6.

4.1 Paul, Faizel, Zak, Idris, and Sam

Eight-year-old Paul was unpopular at his school. He is English and Christian in an ethnically and religiously mixed school. Other pupils explained his unpopularity by characterizing him as unsuccessfully aggressive; teachers also saw him as physically and verbally aggressive. But Paul felt bad about being unpopular.

The playground is ripe for exclusions and establishment of dominance. In Paul's school, the soccer ball was the symbol of power: the rule on the soccer field was that whoever brought the ball decided who got to play. Faizel appeared to be in the position of dominance, although not everyone acquiesced to his exclusions. Paul was repeatedly left out and felt increasingly bad, although he didn't tone down his "bossiness" and competitive and aggressive behavior. In fact, being excluded seemed to make matters worse.

With his teacher, Miss Chahal, an intervention plan was developed that involved helping all the students relate to feelings of being left out. Later that year, Paul told the ethnographer, Ruth Woods that, although Faizel and the other boys had been excluding him, they were recently nicer to him. Paul's explanation for the change was that he had hit Sam, who was notoriously physically aggressive himself. His discussion with ethnographer Ruth Woods follows:

PAUL: Well the thing was after maths he [Sam] started saying stuff like, really horrible, and I asked Sandeep where is he and he said I'm not telling you.

RW: Did he? Why did he say that?

PAUL: Cos he knew I was gonna fight him. I went up to him

RW: [interrupting] How did you find him?

PAUL: I just looked around and I saw him. I went up to him and I said all right Sam and I just went whack! (Woods 2013, 69)

Woods remarks that "later in the interview, Paul commented on the fact that his teacher's interventions had not helped his situation. I had just asked Paul how he felt after he hit Sam" (Woods 2013, 69).

PAUL: I wasn't really happy about it, but I had to do it. When I ask Miss something it never works really.

RW: Do you think it could've worked if Miss Chahal had done something different, or do you think it was just impossible to sort it out that way?

PAUL: It's impossible to do it the way Miss Chahal said. I won't punch anybody else. If Sam does it again really bad for another couple of months I'll do it again. (Woods 2013, 69).

Paul's efforts to become popular heightened as a result of his physical fight with Sam, and future physical aggression served to situate him in a position of more dominance as well as increased popularity. Paul learned that, admonitions not to harm others to the contrary, physical fights are very efficacious in gaining dominance and status (Woods 2013, 70). The question that teachers and psychiatrists face is: how concerned should they be about the development of Paul's aggressive and defiant behavior?

Aggression is not the same as defiance, but sometimes they go hand-in-hand. Sometimes behavior is misunderstood as aggressive when it is not quite that clear. And some kinds of aggressive behavior may count as objectively "good." In this chapter, I present the current thinking on forms of aggression. My analysis will reveal that the concept of aggression is unclear yet, at the same time, overly simplistic. The implication of my literature review is that, when the construct of aggression is used to identify children who might have ODD, it does not clearly pick out any one kind of behavior. To hark back to Chapter 1, Section 1.1, on a Wittgensteinian notion of family resemblances, different types of aggression are family resemblances. As with the medical kinds of patient rights and clinician responsibilities discussed in Chapter 1, the various types of aggression are family resemblances because the kinds of things they are do not have categorical and definitive boundaries. A related concern that emerged from my literature review is that little discussion exists as to what makes some types of aggression or defiance wrong. Chapter 5 takes up this question more thoroughly, but this chapter provides the basis for seeing how complicated such an answer would need to be.

4.2 Aggression, oppositional defiant disorder, and conduct disorder

One of the most common reasons why children and adolescents in the United States are referred to mental health clinics or treatment centers is that they fail to comply with developmental norms for good behavior. In other words, many of these children show aggressive and antisocial behavior—a pattern associated with ODD and CD (Frick and Ellis 1999). Frick and Ellis say that it is this kind of misbehavior that raises the greatest degree of social concern, because it can involve intentional and direct harm to others (Frick and Ellis 1999; see also McEachern and Snyder 2012). Not all aggressive and socially disruptive behavior signifies a developmental pathway toward mental disorder; but Antisocial Personality Disorder and psychopathy, including egocentricity, callousness, manipulativity, impulsivity, irresponsibility, and antisocial behavior, are serious outcomes to consider (Frick and Ellis 1999, 147). Again, not all disruptive and harmful early behavior results in later violent criminal behavior, but violent adult offenders often have early childhood histories of antisocial and aggressive behavior (Frick 2006, 311). Thus, an understanding of the construct of aggression is both medically and socially important.

All children face the developmental task of building a knowledge base of necessary skills for navigating their way through the world. These skills include learning to read and write, being able to hold a conversation, being able to think critically, and being able to behave in ways that aren't harmful or annoying to others. These norms contain positive values in that they aim to help individuals compete, succeed, and flourish, and to provide "glue" for social groups. Thus, norms serve the function of encouraging education into reading and writing and fostering basic civil behavior. Given such developmental tasks, one can see why the indignant but amusing children's exclamation "You're not the boss of me!" might become less charming in children who see themselves as equals to adults or who exhibit a drive to defeat adult authority. However, a rejection of adult authority is not enough to worry adults about the potential development of aggressive and defiant behavior in children; after all, exaggerated defiance is often a normal part of a child's attempts to separate and individuate from authority (Frick 2006). Behavior that is considered oppositionally defiant is characterized as "a frequent and persistent pattern of angry/irritable mood, argumentative/defiant behavior, or vindictiveness, persistent stubbornness, resistance to directions, and unwillingness to compromise, give in, or negotiate with adults or peers" (DSM-5 2013, 463). Children who receive this diagnosis or one of CD are considered negative, defiant, disobedient, and hostile toward authority (Loeber et al. 2000, 1469). They are grandiose, in that they think themselves smarter than adults, and use strategies such as guile, cunning, and lying to manipulate others, seeming not to feel an obligation to be fair (Riley 1997). They disrupt social situations and victimize others, violating others' basic rights and defying social norms and rules (Loeber et al. 2000, 1469). In sum, many of these children are viewed as socially disruptive, highly impaired, and unlikely to get better. However, the prognosis is poorer with respect to children with CD than those with ODD; most children with ODD do not develop symptoms of CD (Blair, Leibenluft, and Pine 2014).

Multiple causes can be identified in children who develop ODD or CD (Frick 2006). Brain dysfunctions have been proposed as one causal pathway. For example, current research on CD suggests that neurocognitive difficulties due to dysfunctions in various parts of the brain give rise to three of its clinical manifestations: deficient empathy, heightened threat sensitivity, and deficient decision-making (Blair, Leibenluft, and Pine 2014; see also Blair 2013, Frick et al. 2014a). Genetic and environmental risk factors must be considered as well. Behavioral problems appear to have moderate-to-high heritability, and both genetic and environmental factors interact with neural pathways (Blair, Leibenluft, and Pine 2014; see also Waller, Gardner, and Hyde 2013). Since ODD and CD are characterized by repetitive defiance of legal, social, and moral norms, children who exhibit such behavior can be said to become dispositionally defiant—that is, exhibiting a trait rather than a state. Traits are thought to comprise the basic structure of personality (Pervin 1994).[1] A trait suggests an enduring tendency to react to many situations in a consistent manner, whereas a state suggests a temporary or passing behavior or emotional response (Endler and Kocovski 2001; Pervin 1994). A state can also refer to a set of symptoms that appears but may abate fairly quickly (Reich 2007). States can pass into traits just as, in virtue theory, repeated actions can develop into virtues or vices over time. Traits may be caused by an interaction between brain and environmental dysfunctions and, thus, behaviors that exhibit ODD or CD are believed to be, or to become, entrenched in personality.

Blair, Leibenluft, and Pine (2014) identify prenatal risks such as maternal smoking or diet that affect fetal development of neural structures. Other environmental causes of ODD or CD must be considered as well. For example, traits may develop primarily as a result of neighborhood and social conditions. Experiences of racism and discrimination contribute to difficulties in school, resulting in low self-esteem and sometimes developing into externalizing behaviors (Pachter and Coll 2009; Brody et al. 2006). The vast majority of Black children live in low socioeconomic conditions, conditions which are correlated with a poorer quality of schoolwork. Poverty is a by-product of inequality that redirects Blacks away from mainstream society (Western 2006, 87); poor education and ill-preparedness for school advancement are consequences of systematic poverty. Frustrated by poor performance and lack of access to good nutrition and adequate health care, and by the continuing impact of historical violence against Blacks (such as transgenerational trauma, double consciousness, and internalized oppression), some children may develop a heightened sense of living in a hostile environment that holds little hope of success for them (see also Western 2006, chapter 4). Defiant behavior, under such conditions, might indeed become maladaptive to success. That is, environmental stressors may be so great that some children develop managing styles that are dysfunctional and become dispositional. But let me be clear, these potential causes of ODD or CD are not only found in some Black children. Wide-ranging maladaptive effects of stressors are found in many children who live in poverty, for white children as much as for Black children. Such stressors also affect children whose parents are migrant workers, immigrants, drug users, or otherwise live in adverse conditions. Some of these children might externalize anger, frustration, and low self-worth in ways that are maladaptive and become traits. Research suggests that a hostile attributional bias and heightened anxiety and aggression in response to frustration or threat are correlated with changes in the normal function of the amygdala, thus locating the defiant behavior found in children with ODD or CD in brain dysfunction (Blair, Leibenluft, and Pine 2014; Crowe and Blair 2008).[2] But, as I will argue, defiance also is complicated for many minority and immigrant children because discrimination, stereotyping, and expectations for following dominant behavioral norms may shape not only the behavior of children—who sometimes are subjected to unfair and biased treatment—but also predictions of dysfunctional behavior.

Consider the childhood-onset subtype of the callous-unemotional (CU) personality dimension. It is "characterized by a lack of guilt, lack of empathy, and lack of emotional expression" (Frick 2006, 315). Frick suggests that these CU traits are similar to those of psychopathic adults. Thus, developmentally, this research suggests a distinct temperamental style (Frick 2006, 317).

> [CU] leads to impulsive and overactive behaviors in early childhood that gradually develop into more defiant and argumentative behavior as a child becomes more verbal and his or her goal-directed behaviors are frequently frustrated by parents. Furthermore, the child's inability to pause and reflect on the consequences of his or her actions, and the inability to perceive the distress caused by his or her actions in others, leads to deficits in the development of empathy and guilt, providing a direct conceptual link to the psychopathic characteristics shown by adults. (Frick and Ellis 1999, 155)

The CU subtype of CD is considered a relatively stable personality trait and has more serious consequences for both the child and others (Frick et al. 2014b; Blair, Leibenluft, and Pine 2014). Children who exhibit CU, therefore, are cause for social and psychiatric concern. Yet I do worry about the science behind some of the studies for CU traits. For instance, delinquent youth were tested for emotional reactions to words with negative emotional connotations, and those with high levels of CU traits showed reduced emotional responses. But among the words chosen to detect CU traits were "gun" and "blood" (Frick 2006, 318). Those words can have a particular cultural currency and resonance for some children: at a meeting with the Black community in my city concerning at-risk youth, children described sleeping directly under their windows so as to avoid getting hit by bullets from drive-by shootings. Living with violence is an everyday occurrence for them and, as such, is normalized. While I am reporting anecdotally, I would expect that this experience is found throughout the nation in many poorer Black (and other) neighborhoods (see Hedges and Sacco [2012] for a depiction of the effects of poverty on people in America). Therefore, it is not surprising that some Black children would respond with little affect to words such as "gun" and "blood." For some children, such responses might indicate the CU subtype of a personality trait of CD; for others, however, I think we need a more complex explanation that includes a cultural analysis. As this chapter unfolds, I will show that in understanding developmental pathways to criminal or mentally disordered behavior, it is crucial to attend to intersections of gender, race, and class when researching, theorizing, and clinically responding to aggressive behavior. When we overlook children's formation and understanding of social identities, positions of privilege and disadvantage, and their struggles for recognition, advantage, status, and domination (hegemony) within their particular milieus, we may make mistaken assumptions and generalizations about aggressive and apparently antisocial behavior instead of grappling with some difficult questions. In particular, embedded assumptions about gendered and racialized norms for dealing with anger, aggression, and rejection can lead us to overlook the possibility that some defiant and seemingly aggressive behavior in children may be a healthy struggle against authority or local playground norms. Furthermore, some behavior that is interpreted as defiant may be culturally inflected and thus misunderstood. The task of interpreting children's defiant behavior is daunting—and potentially clouded with stereotypes (see Box 4.1 for further explanation of stereotypes).

Let me stress that I am not arguing that problematic and dysfunctional children's behavior is only a matter of subjective representations and interpretations. I do believe that some children display behavior that fits the current criteria for ODD or CD. I am pointing out unnoticed or more hidden factors in children's developmental lives that make children's personality characteristics more difficult to understand or determine clearly. The first step is to present various distinctions found in my literature review and to explain how these distinctions render the construct of aggression unclear.

Box 4.1 Understanding stereotypes and stereotyping

The language of a "stereotype" arose in the late eighteenth century in the context of the technological development in printing of a mold that provided a uniform cast (Gilman 1985). It developed into an abstract concept that, in its strict meaning, still refers to a template that allows us quickly to categorize things into groupings and to organize the plethora of stimuli bombarding us. Thus, prima facie, a stereotype is neither good nor bad. But the deployment of stereotypes is more complicated than that. Lawrence Blum distinguishes between stereotypes (the noun) as culturally salient entities and stereotyping (the verb) as a cognitive and psychic activity that individuals utilize with respect to groups (Blum 2004). Stereotypes play a crucial role in how individuals think about, feel about, and decide to act toward others (Cudd 2006, 68). Ann Cudd defines them as "generalizations that we make about persons based on characteristics that we believe they share with some identifiable group" (Cudd 2006, 69). Thus, the formation of stereotypes is a type of categorizing. The cognitive act of stereotyping involves a complex series of inferences about characteristics that individuals believe set people in one group apart from people in other groups; as such, they form the foundation of our beliefs about groups (Cudd 2006). Most of us understand stereotypes primarily by their negative connotations. A negative stereotype is a false or misleading generalization that is intransigent with respect to evidence to the contrary. It is a generalizing, fixed, false belief. Stereotypers are "cognitive misers"; they are efficient, intractable, and often wrong generalizers. In other words, stereotypes not only help us make quick and efficient judgments; they buffer us from anxieties and fears by creating an external Other who is "bad" to our "good," and they arise when we perceive that our sense of self-integration is threatened (Gilman 1985, 15–35).

Studies in cognitive psychology give us reason to think that stereotyping is an unavoidable feature of cognition. But, as Cudd points out, much injustice is done to individuals (and to groups) with the application and reproduction of stereotypes in our attitudes and treatment of one another. We tend to favor in-groups and disadvantage out-groups of the stereotype while simultaneously creating and maintaining those very in- and out-groups. The injustice done through stereotyping suggests that stereotyping activity is immoral (Cudd 2006, 69).

4.3 **Frameworks for understanding aggression**

4.3.1 **Overt and covert aggression**

One frequently cited theory is that two forms of early antisocial development exist: overt and covert (McEachern and Snyder 2012). Overt antisocial behavior involves openly hostile and defiant actions, such as disobedience and fighting. Overt antisocial behaviors such as physical and verbal aggression are performed to gain dominance or advantage over another during a hostile (or perceived hostile) encounter. Covert antisocial behavior, on the other hand, refers to activities that are more surreptitious or sneaky in nature, such as lying, stealing, cheating, running away, truanting, and drug use (McEachern and Snyder 2012, 501). McEachern and Snyder posit that covert behaviors are engaged in so as to avoid detection.

4.3.2 **Physical and relational aggression**

A corollary of the overt/covert distinction that is found in current empirical findings about developmental markers for ODD is between physical aggression and what is called relational aggression. Relational aggression is defined as behavior that harms or threatens to harm others' relationships (Crick et al. 2004, 71). Behavior that harms relationships includes threatening to end a friendship unless the friend does what the threatener says, socially excluding someone, giving someone the silent treatment, and spreading hurtful rumors, thus correlating with the kind of aggression identified as covert antisocial behavior. This distinction is widely believed to be gendered, based not only on empirical research, but also on what I believe to be assumptions and norms about masculinity and femininity. According to Crick et al. (2004), boys are associated more with physical aggression or the threat of physical violence—in other words, overt antisocial behaviors—while research indicates that girls are more likely to engage in what is called relational aggression. In the school setting, Putallaz and Bierman (2004) found that teachers and parents rate boys as more aggressive than girls, and surmise that the gender gap begins around age four. As will become clear, I question a simple generalization of gendered differences. Focusing on gender differences in disruptive behavior as an umbrella term, Putallaz and Bierman suggest that "disruptive boys more often hit, push, and destroy things than disruptive girls, but disruptive children of either gender have temper tantrums, argue, talk back, whine, break rules, and refuse to comply with parental requests" (Putallaz and Bierman 2004, 141).

4.3.3 **Direct and indirect relational aggression**

Sarah Coyne et al. (2008) further distinguish relational aggression as either direct or indirect. According to these researchers, direct relational aggression takes the form of overt manipulation, such as threatening to break off a friendship or relationship if the threatened one does not do what the aggressor wants the other to do. Overt aggression is found primarily in young children and in adult romantic relationships. Indirect relational aggression occurs when the aggressor uses circuitous means to hide her or his malicious intent (Coyne et al. 2008, 577). This type of aggression is apparently considered relational because it does not involve physically aggressive behavior but, instead, interpersonal relationships. (Already, we can see that the concept of manipulation is applied in a confusing way; I return to this point in Section 4.3.4.) This leads Coyne et al. and some other researchers (for example, Liben and Bigler 2002; Maccoby 1988, 2002; Fagot, Leinbach, and Hagan 1986) to explain the association between girls and relational aggression in terms of socialized gender norms, as Section 4.3.4 reports.

4.3.4 **Relational aggression and the construction of femininity**

Coyne et al. suggest that the effects of aggression may have more impact on girls because relationships are a commodity they value highly (Coyne et al. 2008, 578). Girls who use non-normative aggression—such as pushing, hitting, and other forms of physical violence—experience more negative effects of their behavior. The greater maladjustment of girls who use physical violence compared to those who use relational violence is due to the repercussions of defying gender norms: "Societal rules dictate that girls should be sweet, gentle, and nonaggressive, unlike their male counterparts who are expected to be confident, assertive, and even aggressive in many cultures where their honor is threatened" (Coyne et al. 2008, 578). Relational aggression allows girls to control relationships and express anger and fear while staying within the prescribed norms for gender characteristics. To a degree, this analysis makes sense: social norms differ for boys and girls, and when those norms are violated, non-rule-followers face name-calling, exclusion, ridicule, and otherwise stigmatizing responses.

In their study of videos of same-gender indirect relational aggression, Coyne et al. (2008) found that the perceivers of boy-to-boy aggression considered the boy's aggression as more justified than girl-to-girl aggression, even though in both cases the aggression was relational and indirect. This finding suggests that, even when girls use indirect relational aggression—thus staying within the bounds of gender norms of femininity—they are judged more harshly than boys who engage in the same behavior (2008). Neither boy-to-boy nor girl-to-girl indirect relational aggression elicited more empathy for the victim, however. Even when the aggression is considered less justified—presumably because the perceivers were drawing on stereotypical norms of girls' aggression—the perceivers in the study did not feel victim empathy.[3]

Other researchers also suggest that the development of gender roles and norms for masculinity and femininity may be important for the development of relational aggression (Liben and Bigler, 2002). The work of Fagot and colleagues (Fagot, Leinback, and Hagan 1986) highlights that physical aggression is decreasing in girls at the same time that gender-role expectations are increasing. It is possible that, in contrast to physical aggression, relational aggression increases among girls as they develop a firmer understanding of female gender roles. Peer-group-specific gender norms may also influence the types of behavior in which children engage (Maccoby 1988, 2002) and the consequences of those behaviors. Crick reports that children who engage in gender non-normative types of aggression (i.e., physically aggressive girls and relationally aggressive boys) are significantly more maladjusted than children who engage in gender-normative aggressive behaviors (Crick 1997). This work suggests that gender norms may be particularly important for understanding the outcomes of aggressive behavior (Crick et al. 2004, 82).

Section 4.3 highlights some of the problems in the current construct of aggressive and defiant behavior. The association of relationality with females is one of those problems. Bosak, Sczesny, and Eagly suggest that a principle of human inference—correspondence bias—is at work, whereby people's behavior is believed to reflect their psychological dispositions (Bosak, Sczesny, and Eagly 2012, 429). This inferential bias leads people to think that women are especially relational and communally oriented because of their social roles. Social role theorists hold that role behavior shapes gender stereotypes through correspondence bias. The findings of these researchers suggest that when men and women are given identical roles, perceptions of sex differences are reduced (Bosak, Sczesny, and Eagly 2012). However, their research does not explain the apparent existence of early relationality in girls (I return to a discussion of children's gender differences in Section 4.5). While I agree that we need to consider the power of gendered socialization in understanding how and why boys are more likely to express anger, hostility, and a need for dominance physically while girls are more likely to express emotions and needs more covertly, I challenge the idea that "nice girls" do not fight and that when we find girls being physically harmful to others, we have reason to believe that those girls have something "wrong" with them: the association of "nice girls" with absence of physical fighting ends up being circular (see Jones

2009b for an extended analysis of Black girls' violent behavior). Furthermore, I believe it is crucial in understanding aggression in children that we not only look at what we take to be gender differences, but also at how the axis of gender intersects with race, ethnicity, and class axes.

More generally, I find the distinctions in the literature on ODD and CD to be confusing and misrepresentative of the social and cultural context of children's play and developing identities. I schematize the various distinctions in order to illustrate this confusion. Figure 4.1 represents what I have inferred.

In addition to the assumption that nice girls do not fight, the various distinctions identified in Figure 4.1 raise other questions. What is the corresponding category to "relational"? If aggression toward others is not relational, then what is its descriptor? Is not physical fighting an activity done between people and, thus, necessarily involving a relationship between at least two people? And isn't the distinction between "direct" and "indirect" (relational) aggression just another way of framing "overt" and "covert" aggression? If so, why should we not just say that overt aggression is direct and covert aggression is indirect? Another question is why we should place only the concept of manipulation under direct relational aggression and not all forms of relational aggression. As I argue elsewhere, the construct of manipulation varies widely and its meaning ranges across a broad domain of behaviors. In clinical literature, it is virtually always pejorative, but what the term refers to is unstable. In social contexts, manipulativity sometimes is built into norms of socially agreed-upon interactive moves, such as between a stripper and her client or in courtship rituals. It also is sometimes praised, as in the emotion management expected of flight attendants (Potter 2006). In addition, when I consider the

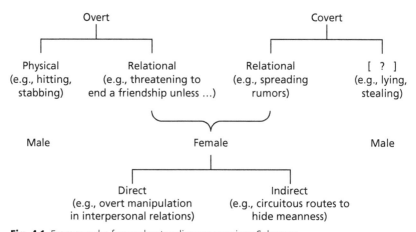

Fig. 4.1 Frameworks for understanding aggression: Schemas.

possibility that most of what is characterized as relational aggression involves some form of manipulative behavior, larger questions emerge: How did the association of relational, seemingly manipulative, behavior with females get such traction? Is it a straightforward matter of empirical data, or are some assumptions and stereotypes about girls and boys lurking in this theorizing? (See Potter 2006.) Finally, does this schema (to the extent it approximates the literature review) hold for all ethnicities and immigrant groups? Or is an assumed "whiteness" at work here?

As indicated, the literature on aggression does not present a clear under-standing of what the content of the construct is or should be. While current distinctions associated with early antisocial behavior may be pragmatically useful (and I'm not convinced they are), they are both under-analyzed and impoverished. For instance, it is not clear what is meant by "lying" or what kinds of lying count as acts of aggression. Is it aggressive to tell a peer he looks good in that cap when the speaker does not think he does—an action that typ-ically is considered a "small lie"? Nor is it clear how "lying" is different from "spreading rumors" or what qualities or properties link "hitting" and "spread-ing rumors." It cannot be that what makes them both aggressive is their hurt-fulness, because not all kinds of hurt to others count as aggression—or, if they do, then the definition seems circular. I cannot sort all of those issues out in this chapter; it would take me too far off the focus of how to interpret appar-ent defiance in children's behavior. I will say, however, that current theorizing on aggression and its predictability for ODD and CD is not sufficient for a complete appreciation for the complexity teachers and clinicians face in inter-preting those behaviors. I say this because the frameworks and distinctions found so far are only part of a matrix of constructions of racial, sexual, and ethnic identities, along with masculinity and femininity, which are negoti-ated through the cultural, ethnic, and class-inflected norms of friendship in schools. As Woods found in her extensive study of children in a large multi-cultural school in West London, "Teachers considered their first and main responsibility to be working out *"what really happened""* (Woods 2013, 185; emphasis added). Physical aggression is easier to determine, because usu-ally its effects are visible on the body of the victim. Even then, the aggressor may be difficult to identify. Less visible acts of aggression—such as spreading rumors, intimidating, or bullying—are more difficult to detect because they are embedded in evanescent temporal communications that can be denied, reframed, and altered.[4]

Sometimes it is nearly impossible to determine the "facts" and, I believe, it can be a misdirected—or at least, an incomplete—goal if teachers and psy-chiatrists try to do so without an appreciation of the complexity of children's playground activities. A main reason to know what occurred and what harms were done is to determine who has been defiant and thus deserves punishment or is so recalcitrant as to need clinical intervention. Sometimes it is necessary to figure out "what really happened" in order to hold kids responsible and to teach them moral and social accountability for actions and consequences. Children do need to learn that their actions have effects both on others and on themselves, but holding children accountable requires that we get it right, as best we can, in terms of justice and fairness.

In Section 4.3, I argued that the construct for aggression is confusing and lacks clarity. In Section 4.4, I present additional reasons to be skeptical about the usefulness of the construct of aggression in understanding defiant behavior. Specifically, I will argue that the construct for aggressive and defiant behavior is not only unclear and under-theorized, but also overly simplistic.

4.4 Situated norms of play, friendship, and harm

4.4.1 Categorizing harms

Norms for harm in the playground seem to be non-legal moral and social ones (see Section 1.2 for a discussion of norms). But the norms that govern default inferences and behavioral responses depend on the dominant schemas of a given context (Haslanger 2014, 29). Sally Haslanger highlights the way that language plays a central role in formulating and activating schemas. Internalized schemas "provide recognitional capacities, store information, and are the basis for various behavioral and emotional dispositions" (Haslanger 2014, 28). As Haslanger explains, these schemas are learned and triggered especially by language; no sharp distinction exists between linguistic meaning and social meaning (Haslanger 2014, 31). She discusses the term "slut," which is a term used to identify features that members within the extension of that term are assumed to have and to guide our responses. Haslanger explains that the norms that govern default inferences and affective/behavioral responses depend substantively on whatever schemas dominate a given context. To call someone a "slut" invokes not only a different population depending on the cultural context, but also how we ought to view and treat members who are presumed to fall within that extensional term (Haslanger 2014). A "slut" is a culturally shaming and socially stigmatizing term that refers to women who are sexually promiscuous; heterosexual men who are sexually promiscuous are not called sluts and are not stigmatized or shamed but, instead, are praised (especially among other men). Among sexually promiscuous gay men, who do call each other or themselves "sluts," the term is used to invoke a schema of pride and liberatory celebration. Toronto was the site of a now-global movement—the annual slut walk—to challenge the sham-ing and victim-blaming language by targeting the slut schema.[5] So, when I think back to Paul's decision to find Sam and hit him for having insulted him (Section 4.1), I might say that norms of not hitting one's peers were overridden by the cognitive schema that Sam's whispered insults invoked. That particular schema, which included whom one could hit and under what circumstances, was triggered when Sam's need to goad and humiliate Paul was put into play, and Paul was responding to schemas in him that allowed him to identify the linguistic meaning of Sam's whispered insults. The meaning-making of insults and responses in that situation was informed and reproduced by local norms in their school and according to the prevailing matrix of class and eth-nic variation there.

It is very difficult to evaluate the status, merit, and content of norms, and much has been written on it (Brennan et al. 2014; see also Nussbaum [1999] for an analyzed example). Here, I comment on the methodology required to understand norms in the playground, in particular, from children's perspec-tives. Once again, I draw upon the work of Woods to query who decides what counts as a harm, whether the children view one kind of norm violation as more serious than another, and why they hold the values they do. This critical analysis raises the question of whose perspective we should adopt in evaluat-ing both the norms of harm themselves and what constitutes violations of those norms. In this section, I will sketch my notion of playground harms, taking into account local norms. I postpone a more substantive analysis of local norms until Chapter 5.

The focus, in this section, is on children and the harms they incur and deliver to their peers. Take Paul, for example. It would seem that Paul was harmed in ways that can make sense of the need he felt to amplify his aggres-sion: he was repeatedly and meanly excluded from playing soccer and from friendship with other boys. But it is not clear that those other boys—Faizel, Zak, Idris, and Sam—violated any norms in excluding Paul or whether or not Paul was warranted in hitting Sam. I wonder, too, how to think about the harms that the other boys inflicted on Paul. To Paul, they were damag-ing enough to call for a response of physical aggression, an act of defiance against the school's norm of not hitting. But Paul's subjective sense that his defiance and aggression were warranted is insufficient to actually establish warrant. These concerns are integrally connected, because often we cannot answer questions of warrant until we know what violation of norms occurred (if any), what those norms were, and what meaning to make of a given viola-tion. I am inclined to think that any hitting by children is wrong. Adults have the responsibility of teaching children that hitting is wrong. As they develop, children still have to figure out when hitting is wrong and why, because adults use physical aggression and force (such as in self-defense), and most adults do not believe that physical violence done in self-defense is a violation of moral norms or norms of civility. But it is one thing to say that children should be held to a norm that hitting others is wrong because we need to teach them to adopt a principle of non-harm, and it is quite another thing to say why children need to learn a principle that many adults do not themselves hold or follow. I am not pointing out an issue of inconsistency or hypocrisy; the issues I am concerned with are epistemological and ethical. To address questions about what norms exist in a particular environ, what the warrant for those norms is, what constitutes a violation of those norms, and when to count a violation of a norm as a serious enough infraction as to warrant punishment or clinical intervention, teachers, parents, and carers need to know more and know well.

Knowing well requires listening and hearing local explanations for norms and, although I make a controversial suggestion here, I add that it requires giving children a degree of credibility.[6] Surprisingly, children sometimes have a clearer moral vision than adults. (See Potter 2001 for an analysis of Dorothy Allison's *Bastard Out of Carolina* [1993] that illustrates this point.) Of course, an investigation into norms of harm and violations of those norms does not end with their testimonies; testing still needs to be carried out to see how their answers extend in temporality and to other habitats (see Code 2008). I develop epistemic, ethical, and pragmatic themes about harms and norms for practical reasoning in Chapter 5; here, I focus on the depth of the problem in making such evaluations.

Woods, for example, found that the children believed that racism was a worse harm than physical aggression (Woods, 2013). Why was that? And were the children onto something important about the relative harms of racism and physical aggression that others of us should pay attention to? The children who held this norm of harm were ethnically mixed; Woods' work raises the question of whether the minority children knew something about the damages done by racism that typically are elided or hidden when privileged, predominantly white adults make evaluative judgments about harms. On the other hand, Woods found that homophobia and its expression received little attention, education, or scrutiny. Teachers were explicit in the moral obligation not to make racist remarks or to behave in racist ways, and children seemed to absorb this message. However, Woods remarks that she never heard a child reporting homophobic epithets or exclusions, never heard an adult reprimand a child for homophobia, and never heard an adult talking to children about it (Woods 2013). So, another question is why homophobic epithets and rejection of peers through invoking "gayness" as a linguistic harm were not counted as violations of any norms in this playground community. It might be the case that the teachers did not think that anti-homophobia on the playground was an important enough norm to be taught. I cannot address all of these issues here. My point is that, in order for teachers and clinicians to make determinations about aggression that is serious enough to merit interventions, they need to engage in the messy and complex epistemological and ethical issues concerning norms and harms. A challenging task indeed. I now return to the topic of types of aggression, adding more characteristics of playground aggression and keeping in mind especially the epistemological challenge of knowing when to be concerned about aggressive and defiant behavior.

4.4.2 Playful aggression

A kind of behavior called "playful aggression" captures one of the great analytic and interpretive challenges to childhood playground interactions. Woods describes playful aggression as "intense, rapid, noisy, playfully aggressive exchanges with their friends: shouting, screaming, insulting or teasing one another, swearing (in English or Punjabi), laughing loudly, and jostling, pushing, chasing or tickling each other" (Woods 2013, 25). She suggests that playful aggression is a way that children negotiate their friendships.

> Amandeep had named Faizel as someone he liked, and when I asked why, he immediately replied, "I just had a fight with him in class!" He explained that Faizel scribbled over his work, so he did the same back, and then they fought, one grabbing the other's neck. I asked Amandeep when he thought that he and Faizel would "make up" from their "fight." He looked surprised and said, "We were just playing about." (Woods 2013, 27).

Woods notes that "playful fights and banter between friends were constitutive of friendship, even when there was some level of physical injury" (Woods 2013, 27). Of course, children who were not competent in banter and playful fighting were marginalized. Different children respond differently to playful aggression, and boys and girls sometimes interpreted playful aggression differently: sometimes boys declared physically aggressive behavior toward girls as "just fun" but the girls experienced it as harmful. These discrepancies make it much harder for teachers and clinicians to hold to one standard of harm. Furthermore, the idea of "playful aggression" presents a conceptual challenge to the construct of aggression overall. What, then, does it mean to call some behavior "aggressive" if not that it distinguishes between harm and play? It sounds right to identify some activities and behaviors as "playful aggression." Consider siblings who are wrestling: they can be goofing around while having an edge of competitive play that carries over into holds so that one gives in. The conclusion I draw is that, when characteristics of aggression are combined with play activities and behavior, the construct of aggression is broadened so as to render it richer but more complex than it currently is.

4.4.3 **Exclusion**

Strategies of exclusion are not necessarily gendered in the way that some research reports. Most studies on exclusion as a form of aggression neglect the role of ethnic differences. Children in several countries have been observed to prefer playmates of their own ethnic group and, in some situations, the dominant group actively marginalizes those from other groups (Woods 2013, 99). Woods' ethnographic study, where the dominant ethnicity of children was Indian, revealed that the outsiders were likely to be non-Indian children: "Indian cultural expertise, such as knowledge of "Indian swear words" and Bollywood films, was a valuable commodity. Those who did not have this knowledge were not able to understand or participate in some interactions" (Woods 2013, 99).

As we have seen with Paul and his peers, some exclusion is intentionally mean and isolating. Exclusion also can occur without malicious intent, and it can emerge without an active excluder (Woods 2013, 95). Children also exclude others on principle, such as to reciprocate a child's racist remarks or to reciprocate a child's excluding behavior by ostracizing the person who is perceived to have been morally wrong. These children's exclusionary behaviors clearly are employing certain norms when they make such determinations, whether or not they do so consciously, but it's difficult to understand how they have arrived at their rules of exclusion. Additionally, given that these children seem to be following certain standards for justified exclusion, it is more difficult for teachers to know when excluding behavior is aggressive, because it is less clear what it even means to call excluding behavior "aggressive."

4.4 **Friendship and loyalty**

Best friends are expected to be loyal. This loyalty takes two forms: the expectation that the best friend will be available when her friend wants or needs her, and the expectation that a best friend shares the enemies of her friend. The demands of loyalty are extremely complex. Zena, for instance, resisted both Maria's and Navneet's demands of loyal playmates, demands which made Zena prickly. Why, then, did Maria and Navneet continue to seek Zena's friendship?

> The girls may have got caught in a vicious cycle. By being unavailable, Zena increased her desirability to Maria and Navneet, so they worked harder to maintain their friendship with her, making themselves more available and hence less desirable

> to Zena. In contrast, because she is not available to them, Maria's and Navneet's feelings of insecurity are likely to increase, leading them, again, to try harder and be more available to Zena. (Woods 2013, 120)

This situation shows the motives and expectations behind the dynamic of exclusions and loyalties in the context of girls' differing needs for independence in the face of possessiveness and assurance. Was Zena toying with her friends' loyalties because of attachment issues, or was she displaying a healthy defiance against norms for consistent sociality? We do not know, but it would be important for teachers and clinicians to understand what motivated Zena because, in order to interpret her sometimes-rejecting behavior as mean-spirited or reasonable, we have to understand more about both Zena's background and the friendship dynamics in this setting. It bears pointing out, too, that possessiveness in this example was sometimes shown by physical proximity and enforced by pushing and pulling—behavior assumed to be the domain of boys.

Section 4.4 gave reasons as to how children's situated and local norms for play complicate the task of teachers and psychiatrists in identifying what counts as aggressive and defiant behavior and when it should be taken seriously. It is not that the norms that children follow are inviolable or should be privileged, but that teachers and psychiatrists might want to be critically reflective about their own assumptions of aggression, play, and harms. Additional reasons to be critically reflective are identified by considering, in further detail, some of the most formative features of children's development. I now turn to consider the process of reproducing masculinity and femininity in the context of other axes of advantage and disadvantage. The discussion in Section 4.5 more fully describes the complex social development of children according to a matrix of race, class, and gender. This discussion paves the way for my analysis in Section 4.6, in which the concept of intersectionalities will illustrate ways that defiance in children may be good, and ways that it may not be defiance at all but just interpreted that way. These sections are meant to show the nuance and complexity that is required for an accurate evaluation of children's behavior as defiant in a clinically worrisome way, defiant in a constructive and healthy way, or not defiant behavior at all.

4.5 Hegemonic masculinities and femininities at work on the playground and in school: Reprise

As Julie Hubbard remarks, it is crucial to attend to cultural differences in how concepts such as aggression, emotion expression, and peer rejection are understood (Hubbard 2001, 1427). Far too little attention has been paid to racial, ethnic, and cultural differences with respect to aggressive and defiant behavior. Because gender is only one axis of social identity, it can provide only an incomplete understanding of aggression and apparent defiance in children. Here I draw on intersectional theory, a theory which emphasizes the ways that patterns of inequality give rise to advantages and disadvantages, privileges and deprivations, depending on one's positionality within those patterns (Collins 1990; Crenshaw 1991). Recall Paul (Section 4.1), whose feelings of abandonment and rejection by other boys in his school, and his responses of physical aggression and fighting, occurred in the context of a mixture of ethnicities. Paul's way of gaining status was to defy his teacher's attempts to stem his aggression by prompting children to care about hurting others' (namely, Paul's) feelings and, instead, to increase his fighting. He had to prove to Faizel—the leader in excluding Paul, and who is a Pakistani Muslim—that he had the "stuff" to merit inclusion in their soccer games and that he was a formidable force if left out. In his case, it worked—at least for a time.

Physical aggression is widely reported to be found in boys as a way of asserting and constructing masculinity (see Woods 2013), but such behaviors are only part of the construction of masculinity. Localized hierarchies have been widely documented in children's peer groups (Woods 2013, 63). Boys experience enormous pressure to display masculinity, in part through acting aggressive and tough. Hence, masculinity is not only constructed in relation to girls; it is shaped and negotiated, often through exclusions and marginalization, through positioning themselves against members of other ethnic groups, who may reject girls in order to move up the hierarchies of masculinity and power (Reay 2001). Diane Reay found that the largely working-class boys in her study, primarily of non-white ethnic identities, jockeyed for positions of status within normative white, middle-class masculinity by positioning themselves against girls. Gee, Hull, and Lankshear (1996) argue that multiple discourses are found in elementary school. They define "discourse" as a symbolic and pragmatic complex exchange that "is composed of some set of related social practices and social identities (or positions). Each discourse produces and reproduces complex relations of complicity, tension, and opposition with other discourses" (Gee, Hull, and Lankshear 1996, 16). Processes of discursive recognition and shifting positionalities are influenced by social class and differing ethnic groupings. Engaging in normative local discourses of masculinity allows boys to gain recognition in opposition to even lower-status groupings, especially including girls. For example, three Bengali boys who were of lowest status within a particular male peer-grouping gained footing by demonizing three middle-class girls. Doing so allowed them to situate themselves discursively as higher status and more powerful through partici-pating in sexist discourse that objectified girls (Reay 2001). The girls' process of constructing femininity must be understood to take place within this con-text of local discourses in a nexus of racialized, ethnic, class, and masculine groupings that also engage in struggles for hegemonic normativity.

Reay's research indicates that "it is the association of normativity with white, middle-class masculinity that seems most difficult for girls to challenge effectively" (Reay 2001, 157). Girls formed into four identifiable groups: "nice girls," "girlies," "spice girls," and "tomboys." "Nice girls" were academically hard-working and behaved well but were viewed particularly by the subor-dinated boys as a contaminating presence on the playground. Being "nice" was a way to conform to norms of white, middle-class femininity and, for working-class girls, "niceness" signified the absence of stereotypical working-class toughness and attitude. The "girlies"—working-class girls, two of whom were white and one Bengali—were actively working to maintain conventional heterosexual relationships by flirting and gossiping about boys and girl–boy relationships. Reay points out that neither of these groups escapes norms of white, middle-class femininity in that girls in both groups aspired to fit in through behavior that conforms to conventional normative femininity: stu-dious or giggly, neither group made waves or challenged authority—including authoritative norms for heterosexuality—or were defiant. The other two groups—"spice girls" and "tomboys"—were both all-white. "Spice girls" were girls with attitude. They exclaimed "girl power!" in ways that sometimes deni-grated boys in hurtful ways. They may have had an advantage in forming their social identities as tough and empowered in ways that girls of other ethnici-ties and working-class girls could not get away with. Still, it's worth noting that these defiant and challenging girls were evaluated more negatively than defiant boys: Reay reports that teachers in the staffroom labeled them as "real bitches," "a bad influence," and "little cows" (Reay 2001). Furthermore, "spice girls," like "girlies," engaged in their share of boyfriend/girlfriend interac-tions. Finally, "tomboys" to varying degrees rejected the notion that they were girls. While this stance might suggest defiance of gender norms and of hav-ing to choose between girlhood and boyhood, Reay notes, and I concur, that claiming to be a tomboy frequently entails for these girls a devaluation of the female world. Jodie, for instance, seems to rail against the status that (most) boys have, yet, in order to do so, she implies that it is best to be a boy:

JODIE: Girls are crap, all the girls in this class act stupid and girlie.

DIANE: So does that include you?

JODIE: No, cos I'm not a girl, I'm a tomboy. (Reay 2001, 161–2)

Thus, Jodie and tomboys like her inadvertently uphold and reproduce the worth and value of males as better than females. The point I want to readers to grasp from Reay's study is that becoming gendered in school and on the playground always occurs in the context of race, class, and sexuality.

Clinicians may wonder why I think this discussion of norms of femininity and masculinity is important to an understanding of when to worry about possible ODD or CD. So that we do not lose sight of the questions, it is important to remember that a necessary part of assessing children's apparently dysfunctional or maladaptive defiant behavior is to understand what to count as defiant, aggressive, and entrenched. My argument has been threefold so far: that theorizing about distinctions in aggression does not yield a clear construct or a dimensional model that is clear; that the focus on gender distinctions has been simplistic; and that a central aspect of understanding violations of norms requires a nuanced understanding of how local norms for playground behaviors are constructed and challenged.

In Section 4.6 I highlight the concerns and complexities of interpreting children's behavior as aggressive by analyzing two populations that are vulnerable to misinterpretation and biased responses: issues that various Black boys face in the school system; and issues that girls of various ethnicities face in school and on the streets. Section 4.6 emphasizes the point that gendered norms and stereotypes always occur in the context of race and class experiences while illustrating how gender norms and stereotypes can shape teachers' and clinicians' understanding of "what really happened."

4.6 **Intersectionalities within Black children**

As I discussed in Section 4.2, school is not only an academic educational institution, but also a socializing mechanism for children. Developmental pathways to socialization or to psychopathology and criminality are affected by school systems' assertions of authority when children are defiant and otherwise hard to manage. Here, I identify cultural factors that affect how children's behavior is interpreted and responded to, looking particularly at racial images and representations. I argue that the norms by which proper development is evaluated are those of the dominant (white, middle-class) group and that they disadvantage other racial and ethnic groups. These institutionalized and systemic attitudes and beliefs negatively affect Black boys' and girls' development and socialization into mainstream society and, therefore, are detrimental to Black people. An examination of these factors may give teachers and clinicians additional reason to be particularly cautious when interpreting children's behavior as dysfunctionally defiant.

There is no question that the anxiety and crushing anguish of daily experiences of racism produce an unrelenting psychological strain (Hines and Boyd-Franklin 1996). Experiences of racial prejudice play a central role in problematic externalizing behaviors, but, at the same time, racial stereotyping and dominant norms for behavior favor interpretations that Black boys are on a path toward mental illness or a life of crime or both. Black girls' development follows a different pathway, with different challenges, as I discuss in Section 4.6.3. When we neglect these matters, we can do damage to ethnic minorities and to societal functioning overall.

Disruptive and defiant behavior cannot be understood outside the context of racialization within a predominantly powerful white population. As Coker et al. (2009) report, 90 percent of Black adults report experiences of racial discrimination. This finding is important because racial discrimination is associated with mental illness. Coker et al. (2009) found that children who reported perceived racial discrimination were more likely to display symptoms of ODD and CD. The question is what those symptoms are indicative of. There are at least three possibilities. Some children and youth do respond to lives of racial discrimination by becoming violent and law-breaking. The question for psychiatry, then, is whether such responses—which pose a danger to others and, often, to themselves—are dysfunctional to the degree that they signify a mental disorder. For others, responses to racism tell us something about the context in which diagnoses are made: that psychiatry is not immune to bias and discrimination and that misinterpretation or misdiagnoses occur. Racism and discrimination are correlated with elevated rates of deviant peer affiliation, violence, anger, and mental health problems in Black youth (Berkel et al. 2009, 2). This is why it is so important to distinguish between behaviors that are signs of genuine mental or criminal trouble and behaviors that are mistakenly read as such and should, instead, be considered as reasonable acts of defiance in the context of racist society. Again, I am not suggesting that unprovoked violence against others be excused but, instead, that interpreting the behavior of Black children and youth in the context of racialized culture is more complicated than some clinicians and teachers may realize.[7]

4.6.1 **Black boys**

A factor that is often overlooked when assessing Black boys who act out in schools is that their low socioeconomic status leaves them poorly prepared for school education and, instead of "feeling stupid," many young boys externalize their frustration and anxiety. Black boys, then, already disadvantaged, are vulnerable to more insidious racism in diagnosis and perhaps in the classificatory system. I pointed out in Section 4.2 that sometimes externalizing behaviors can indicate—or develop into—traits and thus give psychiatrists reasons to intervene clinically. This section illustrates how important it is to disentangle racism as a factor in misinterpreting and misdiagnosing people from racism as a cause of maladaptive behavior that may or may not indicate a mental disorder. Clinicians as well as teachers face the challenge of discerning between maladaptive behavior that may be a response to racism, and the hegemonic production of racial biases that can lead to misinterpretation and misdiagnosis of some minority people's behavior.

Let me elaborate on the issue of bias. Highly stratified societies such as the United States make it difficult for people to perceive the racialized Other without confounding the culturally and socially situated individual with racial bias and stereotypes. A salient example is found in the association of Black males with higher rates of criminality. Blacks are eight times as likely to be imprisoned as whites (Western 2006, 3), and Black males are much more likely than whites to be arrested for a drug offense—and to go to prison if arrested—even though they are no more likely to use drugs than whites (Western 2006, 50). Life milestones such as college graduation, military service, and marriage differ significantly from whites to Blacks, but the greatest inequality is in racial differences in imprisonment (Western 2006, 28). In addition, especially within some Black communities, youth would rather project a "bad" image than a "mad" one because a main barrier to treatment is that mental illness holds a stigma that going to prison does not (see Shelton 2004, 132). These results of the social and legal system are not a result of fair "colorblindness." In *The New Jim Crow* (2012), Michelle Alexander argues that institutional control of Blacks has not decreased since slavery and the Jim Crow laws but, instead, has been transformed from one form into another insidious and damaging racialized method of institutional control. The current method, Alexander argues, is that of mass incarceration of Blacks.

> The adoption of the new system of control is never inevitable, but to date it has never been avoided. The most ardent proponents of racial hierarchy have consistently succeeded in implementing new racial caste systems by triggering a collapse of resistance across the political spectrum. This feat has been achieved largely by appealing to the racism and vulnerability of lower-class Whites, a group of people who are understandably eager to ensure that they never find themselves trapped at the bottom of the American hierarchy. (Alexander 2012, 22)

Megan Kaden comments on the tensions and confusion that the specter of incarceration presents for Black children:

> There is no question that the juvenile justice systems are overpopulated by Black boys: messages from the justice system, the media, the educational system, employers, and federal, state and local governments support the notion that African

Americans are "inferior and troublemakers." Such harmful messages create racial anxiety and fearfulness among African Americans when they must function in mainstream society. The clash of the desire to succeed and the knowledge of the barriers one is up against make the internal psychological and emotional landscape a confusing and often tumultuous one for African American children and adults. (Kaden 2009, 4)

American inequality thus produces a collective experience for young Black men that is wholly different from the rest of American society—a "profound social exclusion that significantly rolls back the gains to citizenship hard won by the civil rights movement" (Western 2006, 6). The stigma of criminality, Western argues, forecloses upward mobility and deflates hope for an entire generation of young Black men with little education (Western 2006, 7). For many, involvement in crime becomes a normal part of economic life (Western 2006, 23); Black adulthood, identity, and masculinity are therefore defined and transformed by the rising risk of imprisonment (Western 2006, 25). Western states that "we should count prisons and jails [and schools] among the key institutions that shape the life course of recent birth cohorts of African American men" (Western 2006, 31).

Black parents aim to socialize their children toward preparation to navigate a racist society while maintaining a conception of the world as a basically good, trustworthy place. They aim to discourage attitudes and behaviors that could be construed as hostile to dominant white society (Berkel et al. 2009). Yet in view of the life trajectory of Black males, it is difficult to see how a tendency to make hostile attributions can be avoided. Consider: in focus groups for Black youth, Black male adolescents reported that "they were less likely to be engaged in the classroom or called on by their teachers and quickly noted that they were viewed as being subordinate to white students, as many underestimated their abilities and their intelligence" and that "their perceptions of being treated less well at school led the adolescents to feel undervalued" (Berkel et al. 2009, 8). Black students routinely experience the classroom as a place where white students are granted more privileges, allowed more leniency in dress, given more credibility in how they address conflict, and disciplined less harshly (if at all) (Berkel et al. 2009, 8). In the United States, Black boys and girls are disproportionately likely to be suspended, referred to law enforcement, physically restrained, or placed in seclusion: one in five Black boys and more than one in 10 Black girls were suspended from school in the 2009–10 school year, according to the Civil Rights Data Collection statistics (U.S. Department of Education 2014; Lewin 2012). Black girls are suspended at higher rates than girls of any other race or ethnicity (U.S. Department of Education 2014). American Indian and Native-Alaskan students are also disproportionately suspended and expelled, but not at as high a rate as Black children, and Asian and white students are suspended the least, based on proportion to population (U.S. Department of Education 2014).

Therefore, with respect to Black parenting, an ideal of racial socialization as instilling self-worth, capableness, and a moral right to fair and equal treatment flies in the face of Black children's experiences within racialized society. Assimilation into white society clashes with students' experiences of unjust and prejudicial treatment, where hostility toward white society may fester but the expression of which endangers their flourishing as they develop.

As this book argues, civility involves "treating others as if they matter" (McGregor 2004, 26) and training children to be civil to others involves socializing them to have the proper attitude toward authority as well as toward their peers. I do not challenge the importance of treating others as if they matter. However, one of the implications of the education of civility is that acquiescence to authority is inculcated in Blacks and called "socialization." Black boys who seem to be defiant and/or hostile are punished for their seemingly disrespectful and open refusal to bow to authority.

We have seen that teachers consider one of their primary tasks as the determination of "what really happened" when playground activities erupt into harm and hurt feelings (see Section 4.3.5). Norms of civility are primarily norms of whiteliness. "Whiteliness" is a term coined by Marilyn Frye (1992) to refer to the complex behaviors that acculturated white people may (usually unconsciously) enact as an expression of their white privilege. "Acting whitely" is different from being white; one can be white and not reproduce attitudes of superiority toward Blacks.[8]

Now, I have claimed that a core aspect of civility is treating others as if they matter, so readers might question why, here, I claim that norms for behavior are whitely: is not civility a universal ideal and not the purview of any particular group? Norms of behavior are whitely when those in privileged and advantaged positions of power are in a position to decide what counts as civility and, thus, how to apply a dominant group's norms for civility to both legal and non-legal domains. The dominant group, with its cultural attributes of whiteness and middle-class home life, are the standard by which the schoolchildren are evaluated and African Americans become Other. "To invest the dominant group's way of life with the stamp of "ideal" or "norm,"" Ann Ferguson writes, "means that the subordinate group's family patterns, language, relational styles are constituted as deviant, pathological, deficient, inferior" (2001, 202). African American boys are praised by their teachers for being obedient and compliant in school even when their behavior does not facilitate (non-ideal) flourishing particular to them. Though the pedagogical message is that all students will succeed according to merit, in truth the racial order of American society is reproduced. Black boys who want to be successful must adopt the mannerisms, behaviors, language, and values of their white peers. Whether this channel is open to them, though, is mediated, in part, by class status. As I indicated in Section 4.2, poverty and lower-class status carries with it reduced access to education in early life, as well as stereotypes about ability and determination to succeed academically. Thus, the sorts of challenges or advantages that some Black boys face in the school system cannot be generalized to "all Black boys." Jockeying for hegemonic masculinity as acknowledged by other Black boys is shaped and informed not only by local cultural norms for masculinity, but also by a particular Black masculinity that seems to offer a bad-boy masculinity as its standard.

Ferguson's study (2001) shows that institutionalized disciplinary practices perpetuate the racial order through disproportionately charging Black boys with defiance (see also Rich 2014). Black boys are sent to disciplinary rooms for behaving in culturally specific ways that then become central to "bad boy" identity formation. Ferguson discusses ""stylized sulking" as a face-saving device" that "involved hands crossed at the chest, legs spread wide, head down, and gestures such as a desk pushed away" (2001, 68). Similarly, Rebekah Denn (2002) discusses African American students' manner of speaking to teachers more as equals than as authority figures because that is how they are treated at home. Such behaviors are taken by teachers and principals to be indications of "bad attitudes" toward authority that warrant detention or placement in Punishing Rooms. Troublemakers, as these young boys come to be known, are "almost by definition characterized by school adults as defiant and disrespectful," where being defiant carries a strongly negative valuation (Ferguson 2001, 69). Both white and Black teachers perceive these behaviors as threatening expressions of a challenge to the demand that students conform to school standards. Teachers read this as a sign that defiant Black students are aligning themselves with lower-class attitudes, and teachers re-assert their authority by sending those students to Punishing Rooms and by predicting criminality and pathology in their futures (2001, 68). These are cases where it looks as if behavior is being misinterpreted in ways that may make diagnoses of ODD or CD more likely.

4.6.2 Defiant girls

I have argued that the development of social identities in children and youth is local, hegemonic, and formed through gendered and racialized tensions. This section focuses on defiance in girls and how clinical interpretations of girls' defiant behavior may focus too narrowly on individual behavior at the expense of discursive formations of shifting social identities in sociopolitical and cultural contexts.

As Kimberley Crenshaw notes, political intersectionality that focuses on antiracist strategies tends to center around Black males. This centering renders invisible the intersectional experience and unique needs of Black women (Crenshaw 1991). As with children on the playground (see Section 4.6), qualities and stereotypes of children in schools are shaped and reproduced in hegemonic struggles. In her examination of the process of producing students as academic and social beings, Joy Lei (2003) argues that stereotypes of and attention to hypersexualized Black males and hyperfemininized Asian/ Asian American females neglects attention to the representation and shaping of Black females and Asian boys (Lei 2003, 159). Once again (see Section 4.6), I call attention to the intersectional ways that social identity and hegemony in children is negotiated, represented, and traversed: the image of Asian boys as "quiet" is contrastively and discursively formed and reproduced in relation to Black boys, white boys, Black girls, white girls, Asian girls, and numerous iterations of ethnic and class positions. In her study, as elsewhere, prevailing images of Black girls are of children who are loud, tough, aggressive, visible, and having "attitude," and the Asian American boys were viewed as quiet.

The work of Nikki Jones (2009a) illustrates how intersectionality emerges when one young woman negotiates street cred with norms of femininity. In this example, intersectional privileges and disadvantages occur in the context of local neighborhood cross-sections of values and expectations of the young woman. Jones describes 22-year-old Kiara as having "light brown complexion and long, wavy hair that suggests a multiracial heritage" (Jones 2009a, 89). Kiara was born and raised in a Black neighborhood and her father was doing time for drug-dealing. As we meet her, Kiara walks the streets collecting signatures to prevent redevelopment of a distressed Black neighborhood. Jones analyzes speech, body language, non-verbal communication, dress, and other modes of everyday social interaction to understand how young women such as Kiara manipulate or violate norms for race, gender, or class. At various points, Kiara shifts the significance of one or another of her intersectional positions; Kiara is aware of oppressive forces that have shaped her and others' lives, and she accentuates similarities or differences as she struggles for survival. This means that she can be pretty, coy, poised, sensual, tough, aggressive, or defiant as she deems necessary in given local situations. As Jones explains, "the shared circumstances of inner-city life engender a shared concern for physical safety and survival. Over time, girls coming of age in distressed urban areas come to realize too how respect, reputation, and retaliation—the three R's at the heart of the [street] code—organize their social worlds" (Jones 2009a, 92). Jones finds that, in the interest of high-stakes survival, girls in the neighborhood strategically choose various displays of gender, race, and class as they simultaneously discursively produce social identity and engage in survival struggles (2009, 92). Kiara thus provides one example of how social hierarchies get reconstituted, resisted, and subverted. Kiara also suggests an adaptive and healthy personality development in that she is aware of varying local norms and expectations and is responsive and flexible in the face of social, economic, and political challenges. Kiara's intersectional identity illustrates a way that defiance can be dispositional and yet healthy: Kiara is dispositionally prepared to behave defiantly when appropriate, but her defiance is not out of control, maladaptive, or entrenched. Jones's analysis of Kiara thus illustrates psychiatric appraisals of psychological health where environmental challenges are met with flexibility and adaptive responses. Such appraisals are contrasted with personality disorders, characterized by a rigid set of responses to environmental challenges.

Readers may be thinking at this point, "This discussion of intersectionality and discursive formations of social identities is interesting, but what does it have to do with aggression and teachers' and clinicians' role in identifying children who may be oppositionally defiant or conduct-disordered?" The point is that aggression is always locally and intersectionally produced or suppressed, punished or ignored, so we need to understand it in a broader context even as we situate it locally.[9] Currie, Kelly, and Pomerantz argue that aggression is constitutive, rather than maladaptive, of dominant culture (2007, 33). Social power constructs girls' agency as a form of aggression, whereas these researchers argue that such a construction indicates a failure to understand girls' agency more generally (Currie, Kelly, and Pomerantz 2007, 23). "Meanness delineated networks and maintained boundaries among girls through discursive acts of ridicule, name-calling, backstabbing, gossip, and "the silent treatment"" (Curry, Kelly, and Pomerantz 2007, 26). It has material effects in that it is both regulatory (it regulates social groupings and membership in friendship circles) and productive (it produces girls' social identities as having or lacking power and agency). As these researchers say, "The harm (and the power) of meanness as an attempt to regulate group membership comes by robbing the "othered" of control over defining "who she is" and "what she is all about"" (Curry, Kelly, and Pomerantz 2007, 26).

Girls' meanness, they argue, is a symptom of a social phenomenon, not an individual one, and these researchers set out to study what meanness means— what it tells us about girls' agency and empowerment:

> Girlhood as a culturally constructed "way of being" is regulated by conventions that girls must be pretty but not "self absorbed" about their appearance; they must be

attractive to boys but not seen to be too sexually "forward"; they must be noticed and liked by the "right people" but not a social climber; independent but not a "loner"; and so on. (Currie, Kelly, and Pomerantz 2007, 24)

Empowerment, as they define it, is "the ability for girls to reflect upon, as a first step in resisting, discourses that position them as subordinate gender subjects. Thus we are interested in how discourses—specifically of social justice—enter into girls' lives" (Curry, Kelly, and Pomerantz 2007, 25). Girls' empowerment is vested in and granted to those who utilize and invoke the rules for middle-class femininity. Girls' own agency is something they try to navigate and negotiate within these constrictive norms of femininity but, as these researchers note, that adults who aim to understand girls' aggressive behavior typically elide (Curry, Kelly, and Pomerantz 2007, 24). Curry, Kelly, and Pomerantz explain that "when a desire for something highly valued (such as social power) cannot be openly expressed (due to the middle-class mandate of "nice-ness"), alternative forms of expression are often invoked" (Curry, Kelly, and Pomerantz 2007, 27). Some girls find themselves in a moral and social double bind, as Vanessa[10] explains:

> You just feel sort of immoral [with the popular kids]. Like [they feel] superior than you sometimes because they have that power. They feel that they can do whatever they want, and say whatever they want. So you kind of feel like you're sort of—like you want to be part of the conversation, but you don't want to let yourself out totally in case you do something stupid, or say something stupid. You know, embarrass yourself. (Currie, Kelly, and Pomerantz 2007, 30)

Local cultures determine "girls' social currency according to whether a girl is pretty, whether or not she is fat, and whether her sexualized self-presentations are "slutty," determinations that are in the hands of her peers" (Currie, Kelly, and Pomerantz 2007, 31). Girls' power comes from their ability to influence the social positions of other girls. But even popularity is not secure, and girls are under constant pressure to maintain or subvert hierarchies of social status and power.

4.6.3 Aggressive and defiant Black girls

In the context of norms of femininity, with expectations for girls that they be nice and relationally oriented, what happens to various cultural norms for Black girls, and how do those norms intersect with normative femininity? Concern about the neglect of the needs and struggles of Black girls that I mentioned in Section 4.7.2 is echoed by Edward Morris, who says that the focus on Black boys and their development of masculinity shifts the experiences of Black girls to the sidelines (Morris, 2007). But, as Morris states, instead of considering the plight of Black boys and girls in the school system together, it is more productive to understand the distinctive ways in which their behavior is viewed as problematic and subject to discipline (Morris 2007, 494). Consider just one example: Danielle Cadet states that Black girls typically were seen as "ghetto" or "loud" for behavior that was usually socially rewarding for their Black male counterparts (Cadet 2013). She reported that Simone Ispa-Landa's study in the context of primarily white suburban schools showed that these boys were welcomed in social cliques but were expected to enact race and gender within constraints of white norms (Ipsa-Landa 2013). However, Cadet notes, "these urban signifiers resulted in the opposite result for black girls, who were seen as "aggressive" and undesirable, with neither the white nor the Black boys showing any interest in dating minority girls. In short, playing out racial stereotypes worked in Black boys' favor, while doing the same was detrimental for Black females."

Direct and overt confrontation are inconsistent with white, middle-class feminine norms; girls who desire to be taken up as feminine frequently draw upon more covert means of expressing anger, resolving conflict, and establishing dominance (Crothers, Field, and Kolbert 2005, 349). For example, "Black adolescent girls may encounter familial socialization practices that proactively prepare them for dealing with oppression, prejudice, and overt and covert discrimination" (Crothers, Field, and Kolbert 2005, 349). As Laura Crothers, Julaine Field, and Jered Kolbert explain, Black girls may use assertiveness in a way that does not conform to white, middle-class standards due to the awareness and knowledge of what it takes to live in a racist world without too deeply internalizing peer negative messages (Crothers, Field, and Kolbert 2005, 350).[11]

Race clearly shapes perceptions of students and teachers' responses to Black students. Studying intersectionalities of race, gender, and class in the classroom, Morris found that many teachers tried to instill in Black girls a white, middle-class ideal of femininity that was docile and, well, quiet (Morris 2007). Teachers are more concerned with teaching Black girls social skills—such as not being "loud"—and worry less about their academic development (Morris 2007). In Morris's observations during a two-year ethnographic study in a public neighborhood middle school, many teachers (not all of them white) saw Black girls as outspoken and confrontational, a challenge to teachers' authority. For instance, one teacher scolded a Black girl for calling out the answer to a problem, presumably because the student spoke out of turn and speaker privileges are something the teacher is to decide, not the student. Other teachers viewed Black girls as disruptive in the classroom, and one teacher described them as "very defiant" (Morris 2007, 503), but Morris's own observations did not agree with their judgments. Morris also did not find the

Black girls "disruptive" in the classroom, even though they sometimes spoke out of turn or talked with one another. Lei argues that loudness is an act of resistance to their Otherness and to their socially proclaimed powerlessness (Lei 2003, 164). The ability to not let anybody "give you any grief" is a survival strategy (Lei 2003, 165). Lei observed, however, that white teachers would walk away from loud Black girls, interpreting their behavior as an aggressive threat. This interpretation reinforced the image of Black girls as threatening and confrontational (Lei 2003, 165). Evaluations of class also influence perceptions, as some teachers interpreted the Black girls' loudness and lack of interactional skills as evidence of poor parenting. Poverty was assumed to be a marker of being lower class, with accompanying stereotypes of the loud, aggressive matriarchal Black woman. In part, stereotypes are at play; in part, rejection of dominant normative femininity.

How should teachers and clinicians think about Black girls who are interpreted and reported as loud, insolent, disruptive, defiant, or confrontational? As I theorized in Chapter 2, civil behavior is one of the aims of social living because it helps individuals and groups cohere and lessens violence. Defiance in the classroom is a case in point—and when students cannot or will not learn the lessons of civility, they can expect to be chastised and even punished. If they still cannot learn lessons of appropriate classroom behavior— especially if their behavior spills out into the playground, the neighborhood, and the family—diagnostic concerns about ODD and CD enter in. My intention, in this chapter, is to disrupt the thinking about that trajectory.

For Black girls, the systematic advantages, protections, and privileges that attach to white girls do not avail. Thus, they need to appeal to alternative survival strategies. Learning to be "ladylike" further disadvantages them because they are required to be docile and submissive even in the face of classroom and playground injustice. Defiance seems a better strategy because it preserves their sense of self and may interrupt the internalization of negative ascriptions and stereotypes. It may be a catch-22 for many Black girls, though, because efforts to ward off the meaning and force of negative ascriptions seem to require that they act in ways that merely perpetuate those stereotypes.

I suggest that a deeper issue is also occurring. In many cases, such as Black girls' "loudness" or confrontational attitudes, the stereotypes are likely to be culturally bound and not mere signifiers of individuals' (or ethnic groups') dysfunctions. Their interactions and behaviors can be tainted by racialized, gendered, and class-based stereotypes. While it is true that a behavior can be culturally inflected and still objectively be problematic, the existence of cultural differences in vocal tone, comportment, assertiveness, and other variants should give us pause: those of us who stand in positions of authority or privilege may interpret behavior as defiant that is an integral part of a student's culture and is not always meant to imply disrespect.

Evidence suggests that the inculcation of white, middle-class norms of femininity is academically bad for Black girls. As Morris reflected about his ethnographic observations, he found that the school he studied put more effort into

> molding Black girls into more mainstream models of femininity—models that included more "proper" behavior such as bodily control and restriction, speaking in a quieter way, and being more receptive to authority and instruction . . . In their genuine attempts to help these girls by teaching them proper ladylike manners, educators often unintentionally stifled the outspokenness and assertiveness that forged academic success for many African American girls at Matthews. (Morris 2007, 509)

Perhaps in order to acquire the requisite academic knowledge and skills, they would do best to resist learning to be ladylike in the interest of achieving school knowledge. The point is that the demand for whitely feminine niceness and quiet not only perpetuates problems in academic development for Black girls, but also entrenches broader social inequalities and injustices that permeate our prison system, our economic system, and our employment system.

4.7 **Conclusion**

4.7.1 **Chapter conclusions**

Defiance and aggression are not the same phenomenon, but are hard to tease apart. This chapter shows that the construct of aggression is complex and messy. It is particularly difficult to apply when evaluating children's conduct because norms for behavior are, to a considerable degree, local and situated. When I also consider intersectional issues, I conclude that, if teachers' primary task is to sort out "what really happened," it is a mighty difficult one. Interpretations of defiant behavior not only require a complex and nuanced understanding of the varieties of aggression and harm, but also a deep appreciation for varying cultural norms in how to behave in the classroom, on the playground, toward one's peers, and toward authority.

Discriminating between internal dysfunction and reaction to social context is exacerbated by racialized norms that often go unrecognized. While I have no doubt that genuinely troublesome behavior exists, I believe that some of it arises out of the messiness of cultural differences and systemic oppressions in hegemonic society. Referring to the looping effect of interactive kinds, Ian Hacking points out that we need to be concerned about "classifications that, when known by people or by those around them, and put to work in institutions, change the ways in which individuals experience themselves—and may even lead people to evolve their feelings and behavior in part because they are so classified" (Hacking 1999, 104). On this view, if young Black boys are being diagnosed with ODD and CD, they may begin to respond to their classification by exhibiting closer approximations to it. Even attempts to defy that classification serve to confirm it. The concern is that schools and other institutions sometimes are not merely identifying an existent mental disorder, but are creating the conditions under which that disorder thrives. Thus, the loopiness of human kinds is one problem that faces teachers who send their students to school clinicians for evaluation. To the extent that ODD and CD are interactive kinds, they are particularly worrisome ones because the diagnoses may get attached to a multiply disadvantaged group.

An additional problem with these diagnoses is that they are vice-laden classifications. John Sadler defines "vice" in the technical sense of meaning acts that are immoral, wrongful, or criminal (Sadler 2014; see also Sadler 2013). He argues that CD is a vice-laden classification by calling attention to linguistic terms found in the criteria, such as "bullying, cruel, stole, destroyed, lies, cons, shoplifting, forgery, truant" (Sadler 2014, 170). One problem with embedded vice-laden concepts is that they fail to distinguish between psychiatry as a caring and curing profession and psychiatry as a form of social control of criminal and moral deviance (Sadler 2014, 172). As I discussed in Chapter 2, the history of psychiatry has collapsed the two, resulting in charges that it is an oppressive and harmful force in people's lives, so it is important to delineate vice from dysfunction when classifying and interpreting aggressive and defiant behaviors. While psychiatric nosology assumes such behaviors to be trait-based dysfunctions, Sadler suggests that they might better be viewed as poor choices or a rejection of prevailing social norms. This latter idea is consistent with what I think is sometimes indicative of good defiance.

The upshot is that, nosologically, the line between normal and pathological defiance is unclear. At the very least, more attention to what the construct of aggression entails is called for. In addition, those who study and fine-tune the criteria for diagnosing ODD and CD need to attend to socially mediated differences such as gender, race, and socioeconomic status in order for clinicians not to inadvertently perpetuate racial and other inequalities in society. The concerns expressed in Section 4.6.1 apply to Black girls as well, although the issues differ. If Black girls respond to stereotyping and subsequent severe suppression of apparently defiant behaviors such as loud and outspoken confrontations with teachers, they may internalize these negative messages and reproduce them. In other words, the kinds of behavior some Black girls exhibit may be interactive ones that damage their academic progress.

The problems I identified in this chapter are not only ones of interpretation or epistemological and ethical challenges regarding analyses of norms. They are also problems for children who persist in being defiant because they believe or intuit that it is better for them. That is, children are not helpless victims of linguistic, moral, and social norms and, thus, cannot help but internalize racist messages or ideologies. Children do think for themselves (more so as they develop, of course). But if the suppressing, punishing, and diagnosing of young Black children who act defiantly are probable outcomes, why would anyone ever deliberately be defiant? As I showed, even appearing to be defiant runs the risk not only of being sent to Punishing Rooms but also of being diagnosed with a mental disorder. Why take the risk?

4.7.2 **Reasons to be defiant**

In this final section, I will offer five responses to the question of why anyone, children included, would risk punishment, retaliation, or even psychiatric diagnosis by being defiant when they are not driven by dysfunctional neural pathways. The first two responses invoke reasons to be defiant that are instrumentally good, while the other three are intrinsically good, although even this distinction is not hard and fast (sometimes our motives and reasons for actions are both intrinsic and instrumental). We have seen that one reason, at least for Black girls, is that defiance of whitely norms may be a way for them to achieve the academic success they need. This reason is instrumental to their achieving a high quality education. Some Black girls may deliberately be defiant because they are aware, to some degree, that it is the only way to deal with the detrimental consequences of racist subjugation in school. Other Black girls may act defiantly based on a similar motive but without conscious awareness of why they are doing so. This, too, may constitute a good enough reason for them to be defiant—although sometimes it is not a reason that they can articulate consciously. Whether or not defiant behavior without reasons should be considered good defiance is a topic taken up in Chapter 5.

The second reason why it is worth being defiant is that behaving defiantly can give hope to the downtrodden, the discouraged, and the underprivileged. Being defiant both expresses hope and, in expressing it, gives one hope—and hope is necessary to survive struggle. As Anthony Reading says, "Hope gives us a vision that things can be better, rather than just continuing as they have been, an expectation that some desired goal can be attained" (Reading 2004, 3).

Having hope leads us to act in ways that we can reasonably expect to bring about a better future. Despair and hopelessness are an abandonment of the future, inculcating a passivity or even destructiveness. (Think about Marie in Chapter 3, whose refusal to attend group activities while in hospital is construed by her therapist as a positive sign of engagement with the world.) Hope is constructively energizing (Reading 2004, 5), and people need that attitude to motivate them to continue to struggle to survive, especially in the face of deprivations, structural disadvantages, and systemic oppressions.

Hope is instrumental to engagement with the world, but unrealistic and overly optimistic hope seems to be foolish or dangerous. Defiant behavior that is either instrumental to a constructive future in general or to a just and quality education in particular must be performed and evaluated in terms of how high the cost will be in the long run. Children need experience to know the extent to which their behavior has consequences that may include long lasting harm to themselves, but a central aspect of development is learning which ways of living bring about advantages—and which bring disadvantages—and to whom, and why it matters that we learn how to think about other people as well as ourselves. Nevertheless, children do develop and, as they do, they may decide that acting defiantly has too great a cost for them. This might sometimes be the most prudent path, but it also opens up the possibility of staying stuck in burdened virtues such as acquiescence, submissiveness, or conformity with oppressive dominating norms. The cost of compromise is also great.

Not all acts of defiance—whether by children or by adults—require such a rigorous costs–benefits analysis. I can think of three reasons why being defiant in given situations is intrinsically good. So the third reason to be defiant is an intrinsic one. The writing of Bernard Boxill suggests that being defiant is good in that it affirms self-respect at those junctions where it might be threatened:

> The powerless but self-respecting person will declare his self-respect. He will protest. His protest affirms that he has rights. More important, it tells everyone that he believes he has rights and that he therefore claims self-respect. When he has to endure wrongs he cannot repel and feels his self-respect threatened, he will publicly claim it in order to reassure himself that he has it. His reassurance does not come from persuading others that he has self-respect. It comes from using his claim to self-respect as a challenge. (Boxill 1995, 102)

Thomas Hill suggests a fourth reason to be defiant, one that I also take to be intrinsically good. Hill's analysis of self-respect includes the value of signaling to others that one has not agreed to give up one's moral rights (Hill 1995). This signaling is something that defiance might do. Moral rights, even from children's perspectives, might include being treated fairly, not being unjustly disadvantaged (meaning not being disadvantaged in systemic and structural ways), and not being interpreted and treated in stereotyped ways. I prefer to frame Hill's point as that of expressing that the defiant individual still expects moral recognition, instead of framing it in terms of rights-talk, but, with that shift, I believe that the idea that self-respect requires moral recognition is an intrinsic reason to be defiant.[12]

Lastly, defiance can indicate—without any appeal to moral rights or assertion of one's basic worth—that some ways of behaving are simply beneath one (Hill 1995, 119). This, too, takes defiant behavior to be intrinsically good in some circumstances. Defiance allows the defiant one to maintain some sense of integrity in the face of perceived unfair treatment. Lynn McFall, in analyzing integrity, argues that, although many or most of our commitments are defeasible, there is at least one commitment each of us holds (or that most of us hold) that is unconditional. According to McFall,

> there is some part of ourselves beyond which we will not retreat, that some weakness however prevalent in others that we will not tolerate in ourselves. And if we do that thing, betray that weakness, we are not the persons we thought; there is nothing left that we may even in spite refer to as I. (McFall 1987, 12)

McFall's idea of unconditional commitments suggests that one reason to be defiant (for children and for adults) is that it preserves a sense of self that is tenuous at best for many disadvantaged or discriminated-against children and adults. Barbara Herman argues that "if we do not care enough about ourselves, we may become less able agents . . . we may also undervalue our happiness by exaggerating the nature and extent of moral requirement" (Herman 2004, 101). Our own happiness has epistemic value, in that if we are unable to enjoy life, we may also have difficulty making wise choices for ourselves or good judgments about others. Sometimes concern for oneself is required as a priority over the needs of others (Herman 2004, 101).

I recognize that, even in cases where defiant behavior seems to be intrinsically good, it may not be wise in the long run: the costs may be too high and the burden too heavy. Sometimes it is too much to expect that it is better, all things considered, to be defiant and preserve self-worth, moral recognition, or integrity. Tessman gives an achingly poignant analysis of ethics and moral reasoning in ordinary living under non-ideal conditions. Moral life, she argues, is fraught with "impossible demands" which make moral failure inevitable (Tessman 2015, 44). Non-negotiable principles, such as integrity seems to demand, may create another moral failure for the person being defiant. So when is it worth being defiant? When is defiance an expression of a bad character trait? In Chapter 5, I take up the question of bad defiance and give reasons as to what constitutes an excess of defiance, why, and what sort of reasoning defiant people can use. I develop a working model of reasoning that undergirds defiance while allowing defiance to maintain a quality of being untamed and undomesticated to some degree.

Chapter 5

Bad and good defiance: Practical reasoning as guide

The public and the media have a keen interest in understanding the kind of person who would violate positions of trust and power, defraud others, and successfully escape the power of regulators, yet appear indifferent to the financial, psychological, social, and familial effects their behavior has on others (Babiak, Neumann, and Hare 2010, 175). There are good reasons to be concerned. Studies indicate that people who are successful in the corporate and financial worlds are often able to rise to high positions of power due to their ability to make persuasive arguments and charm others with friendly and engaging interactions—qualities that look an awful lot like features of psychopathy: callousness, grandiosity, and manipulativity (Babiak, Neumann, and Hare 2010, 176). In fact, some people who score very high psychopathy ratings are considered to have great potential to hold senior management positions (Babiak, Neumann, and Hare 2010, 189). This is not to say that people in high positions in corporations and finance are psychopaths but, instead, that they may show features of it (e.g., deception and lying, callous and ruthless use of others). What it does suggest is that people are rewarded in the corporate and finance worlds for features and skills that are considered to be part of psychopathy.[1]

I start with the story of a white American male who caught the public's attention when a popular book was written about him. The man, Christian Gerhartsreiter, seems to characterize both financially rewarded psychopathic characteristics and criminal—perhaps clinical—pathology.

5.1 The Man in the Rockefeller suit

In the early 1980s, young Christian Gerhartsreiter immigrated to the United States to become the person he was not able to be in his native Bergen, Germany. Over the next few decades, Christian would changes identities several times, charming friends and acquaintances, and ultimately being admitted to the highest echelons of society. He accomplished this by adding greater and greater embellishments to his history and social connections, ultimately claiming to be related to the wealthy and influential Rockefeller family. He exhibited social poise and exercised what I would call "impression management" as he climbed the social ladder. Gerhartsreiter's alleged social standing merged with actual social and financial status via his ability to con others into giving him enormous amounts of money, thus allowing him to support an increasingly luxurious lifestyle and simultaneously sustain the image of himself as a Rockefeller. He was eventually caught when he kidnapped his young daughter during a divorce and, several years later, was convicted of murder.

How did he manage to pull off this series of cons and deceptions for as long as he did? To what extent was he engaging in criminal acts? It is clear that kidnapping and murder are morally wrong, criminal acts. (This is not to say that "morally wrong" and "criminal" necessarily are conjunctives; for instance, most people take lying to be morally wrong but not criminal, and flagrant rudeness to be morally offensive but not criminal.) Gerhartsreiter clearly was defiant of common-sense moral and legal standards, and his behavior seems to call for explanation. Clinicians and laypersons might regard his persistently defiant behavior as a sign of a psychopathy—specifically, Antisocial Personality Disorder (ASPD).

Patients with ASPD seem to epitomize bad, or vicious, defiance. They defy the law, disregard moral norms for regarding others as intrinsically worthwhile, and flaunt standards for truth-telling. Gerhartsreiter, therefore, presents a case study in defiance gone wrong. But how, and why, exactly? In this chapter, I first raise questions about defiance by looking at the signs and symptoms of ASPD, and I then examine those questions by considering qualities and characteristics that defiance as a virtue holds. I propose an account of some of the features of practical reasoning that will assist readers in distinguishing between good and bad defiance. The theory of defiance as a virtue developed in my book thus far will be filled out in this chapter in a way that clarifies what is wrong with antisocial behavior, so as to identify constraints on counting defiance of the mentally ill as a virtue and to indicate what defiance as a virtue would look like.

The issue I examine is what qualities or characteristics would make defiant behavior wrong and why. To answer such questions, it is not enough to point to broken laws, as the laws themselves may not reflect the virtues needed for flourishing. Furthermore, my claim throughout this book has been that sometimes defiant behavior should be seen as virtuous. My defense of defiance thus seems to allow for lawbreakers sometimes to deserve praise, not prison. Gandhi's defiant action of publicly burning his pass in South Africa is an example of praiseworthy law-breaking, because the law itself was fundamentally damaging to Black South Africans. Should the behavior of those with ASPD be counted as a kind of protest? Civil disobedience? Defiance? This chapter begins with a look at ASPD as a starting point for answering larger questions about the line between good and bad defiance.

5.2. **Antisocial personality disorder**

Psychopathy has many historical monikers: moral insanity, degenerate constitution, congenital delinquency, psychopathic personality, and ASPD. All of these terms are used pejoratively and call up negative images of people (Oglaff 2006, 520).

A look at the characteristics in criterion A of ASPD (see Box 5.1) gives an idea of why people who fit these symptoms are disparaged. The social norms, disciplinary functions, and moral psychology of those in communities and

---

Box 5.1 **The diagnostic criteria for ASPD**

A. A pervasive pattern of disregard for and violation of the rights of others, occurring since age 15 years, as indicated by three (or more) of the following:

  1. Failure to conform to social norms with respect to lawful behaviors, as indicated by repeatedly performing acts that are grounds for arrest.

  2. Deceitfulness, as indicated by repeated lying, use of aliases, or conning others for personal profit or pleasure.

  3. Impulsivity or failure to plan ahead.

  4. Irritability and aggressiveness, as indicated by repeated physical fights or assaults.

  5. Reckless disregard for safety of self and others.

  6. Consistent irresponsibility, as indicated by repeated failure to sustain consistent work behavior or honor financial obligations.

  7. Lack of remorse, as indicated by being indifferent to or rationalizing having hurt, mistreated, or stolen from another.

B. The individual is at least age 18 years.

C. There is evidence of conduct disorder with onset before age 15 years.

D. The occurrence of antisocial behavior is not exclusively during the course of schizophrenia or bipolar disorder. (DSM V 2013, 659; see also Hare and Neumann 2009, 792).

societies help to regulate and inhibit behaviors that threaten to damage the fabric of groups. Norms of civility, as I argued in Chapter 2, work as a kind of social glue that holds together authoritative bodies and subjects in their various roles, jobs, skills, needs, and interests. Some system of governance, justice system, and educational and medical/psychiatric infrastructure seems necessary to point people in right directions and away from danger. Qualities of character such as empathy, a disposition to value personal ties and unknown others, the ability to forgive, to feel guilt and remorse, the capacity to identify moral wrongs and to try to avoid them, and to fear punishment, seem to be worthy of value. Yet the very idea of society being a fabric of interwoven threads and textures is a metaphor that disguises the ways that fabrics are artifacts whose elements are composed of various strengths, knots, and twists and often are compressed, warped, stretched, and ripped. Throughout the book, I have emphasized the reality that societies are organized in ways that damage and oppress some in ways that benefit others and that demand conformity and that fail to understand, or medicalize, those with social stressors, psychiatric needs, or practices different from the expert or authoritative body. ASPD thus illustrates the challenges of determining when defiance is a vice and when a virtue—or neither, if the defiant behavior is involuntary.

The behaviors identified in criterion A of ASPD as symptoms of mental disorder are even more difficult to evaluate when set in the context of racialized societies. In Chapter 4 I analyzed a matrix of advantages and disadvantages that intersect with children in multiple ways and argued that a clear construct does not emerge for aggression and defiance in the clinical or educational domains. I noted potential biases and stereotypes at play in evaluating and responding to defiant behavior in children. A similar pressing concern is found in the research and application of diagnostic measures of ASPD. The meta-analysis done by Skeem et al. (2004) found that academic research identifies individuals of African descent as significantly more likely to be psychopathic than individuals of European descent. However, their own research debunks such ideas. They note that criminal justice and public policy are likely to be driven by public perception of "the crime problem" and its causes. As such, it does not bode well for minorities that the public already seems to be predisposed to viewing them as more psychopathic than the majority. Their research strongly suggests that prejudices and stereotypes are at play in the medical and criminal justice systems as well as in social media and public perception. It also raises central philosophical questions about relative and objective norms for reasoning, morality, and civility.

So, it is unclear when defiance is good and when it is bad. Some people, whether through trait or state fault lines, or an interaction between them, behave in overwhelmingly egocentric ways and are violent toward others, impulsive, and controlling; they exploit the vulnerable to achieve power and intimidate others to control them (see Hare 2013). In order to understand what makes the behavior of people with ASPD or antisocial tendencies bad or wrong, we need an understanding of harm that addresses what is wrong with being deceptive, exploitative, or physically aggressive. Although I do not offer a full theory of harm, I set out what I consider to be some of its main constituents.[2] The perspective from which harms are evaluated will affect a theory of defiance: if authoritative harms against oneself are great enough, one might be impelled to defy authority, but the subjective experience of harm is not always a reliable method for determining when to be defiant or when to worry about others' mental status. To address this problem, I discuss norms of practical reasoning, a relaxed version of *phronesis*. I do so with some hesitation; as I argued in Chapter 3, the passion and unboundedness of defiance has value and merit, and an account of reasoning well is likely to tame and tether it in ways that tarnish this important feature of defiance. Therefore, my aim is to clarify what goes well when defiance is good and what goes wrong when defiance is bad by giving an account that attends to good enough reasoning and that entails passion and affect as well. I will argue that the ideal for virtuous defiance occurs when defiant behavior a) arises out of a response to basic or egregious harms such as oppression or injustice; b) is self-preserving; c) expresses at least some features of practical reasoning; d) expresses a mean for affect and passion; e) is done from a dispositional state; and f) does not contribute to harms that are themselves oppressive or unjust, or at least that it does not contribute to unjust or oppressive harms any more than other actions that we deem ordinary and relatively acceptable—such as eating meat, or wearing clothing that was produced through exploitative conditions, or exhibiting implicit bias against Blacks when one stands farther away from them in the elevator.[3] These conditions for virtuous defiance are themselves normative and, as such, are open to challenge and negotiation. It assumes that we can get it wrong about when, or whether, defiance is reasonable, justifiable, or a good way to be. Additionally, virtuous defiance, in this domain, is sometimes a burdened virtue and sometimes not (see Chapters 2 and 3). As I explained in Chapter 3, when defiance is a virtue, it may be a lighter, but still burdened, virtue—because it is done under conditions of disability, oppression, or structural disadvantage, it may not be a "pure" virtue. But I also hold that some defiance is unburdened, in the sense of Tessman's Trait v_1: it sometimes is partly constitutive of living well enough.

The specific questions that arise at this point in the book are these: What status do ethical claims of accountability have, and to whom are we accountable? How can we assess when another person or patient has a good enough reason to have violated a norm? In particular, what norms of practical reasoning can we draw on in judging a person or patient's defiant behavior as reasonable—that is, good and beneficial—or bad and harmful? What warrant do we have for holding some norms of harm as serious enough infractions to punish, criminalize, or medicalize? How can people themselves reason well (or well enough, at least) about being defiant? I take up these questions in Section 5.3.

I will argue that defiant behavior needs to be justified on more than solely subjectivist grounds, and that good practical reasoning is a guide to providing such justification.[4] I am using the term "justification" not as a strong demarcation from "explanation" but as connoting something more like "can be endorsed," "is defensible," or "can provide sufficient reasons for." By saying that defiant behavior cannot only be justified subjectively, I mean that a subjective sense that one is justified in behaving defiantly is not sufficient to justify such behavior. On my view, good practical reasoning eschews the subjective/objective dichotomy—or, to put the point differently, good practical reasoning expresses both subjective and objective features. Nevertheless, as I have argued, a person or patient's assessment that defiant behavior is called for needs to be taken seriously and not merely regarded as symptomatic. Practical reasoning does place constraints on how far one can extend justification for a subjective sense that defiance is called for, but because practical reasoning is normative, and norms themselves always are socially mediated, judgments "from the outside" need to be engaged critically and not just assumed to be justified themselves. Therefore, the account given in Section 5.3 of practical reason is just a guide, a heuristic, for judgment and not an argument for necessary and sufficient conditions.

5.3 **Practical reasoning**

In this section, I concern myself with practical reasoning as it applies to the process of deliberating about behavior or evaluating the behavior of others. I set out features of practical reasoning[5] that would allow people to evaluate when it is done adequately with respect to defiant behavior. Again, I am not claiming that these are necessary and sufficient reasons for practical reasoning.

In focusing on local norms, as I have in Chapter 4, I raise the specter of a crisis in the foundations of ethical reasoning. Universalist accounts of ethics historically were justified on external grounds such as metaphysical ones. As I noted in Chapter 2, Aristotle holds that the metaphysical essential nature of human beings as rational requires virtues of character and of thought. That conception of ethics was rejected on the grounds that a metaphysical or naturalist account of such conceptions cannot be justified. Later, only particularist, subjective ethics was accepted, with its justification grounded from within a given tradition or practice: If no external metaphysical or natural grounds for justification exist, then particularist ethics can be justified internally only. But, then, both universalist and particularist, local ethical norms are arbitrary—not based on any external objective grounds (O'Neill 1996). As Onora O'Neill argues, a vindication of ethical claims cannot be based on the "demands" of some supposed idealized or transcendent reality, or on the characteristics of particular agents, or on the features of certain social practices or institutions (O'Neill 1996, 125). While I depart from O'Neill on her universalizability method for determining justice, I draw on her work to identify some of the important features of practical reasoning.

5.3.1 Inclusivity: From particularities extended

O'Neill's aim is to construct an adequate account of practical reasoning that does not rest on pre-emptive metaphysical or unjustified starting points and that allows for—indeed, requires—both particularist and universalist practical reasoning. The aim of practical reasoning, on her account, is to guide action in ways that fit the world, to some extent, to its recommendations and not the reverse (O'Neill 1996, 42).[6] She defends a universalist account of justice and argues that particularists often collapse some important analytic distinctions.

Some critics of universalism think that any abstraction from particularities results in an elision of differences. O'Neill points out that abstract principles are a necessary feature not only of ethical reasoning but of thinking itself. Abstract principles per se are not a quality of reasoning that can be avoided. I would add that abstract thinking does not require that we bracket off affect. Indeed, I eschew a sharp reason/emotion dichotomy and follow Alison Jaggar in holding that emotions have epistemic value (Jaggar 1989). In this, I differ from Tessman who emphasizes the role of intuition as distinct from reason (Tessman 2015). With respect to practical reasoning in ethics, O'Neill's thinking is that principles do abstract from difference, but they need not deny particularity and diversity (O'Neill 1996, 77). Indeed, we need to abstract from the particularities of given locales, epochs, and situations in order to construct ethical reasoning that avoids subjectivism and relativism. Expanding outward from particularities and local domains, we reach a degree of uniformity. That uniformity, however, does not fix the content of ethical reasoning. By this, O'Neill means that even while universal principles prescribe some degree of uniformity (such as "do not enslave others"), they under-determine the action, allowing for diversity. As Margaret Walker puts it,

> moral understandings include shared norms, principles, maxims, and guidelines . . . we must also for example, understand when and to whom standards apply, by whom and in what cases they may be credibly invoked, what they require or leave to the discretion of particular people in actual situations, and what assessments and costs attach to their fulfillment or disregard. (Walker 2007, 237)

Walker thus points to issues of authority and domain that a good enough process of practical reasoning would need to address.

5.3.2 Domain specificity

Jennifer Morton says that the normative force of particular or local norms requires explanation; particular norms cannot merely be subsumed, ignored, or rejected. "The conditions under which it makes sense for an agent to guide a particular norm in her deliberation are sensitive to contingent environmental conditions the agent is in" (Morton 2010, 570). One of the norms of rationality that Morton discusses is the Stability Norm. This norm holds that a reasonable person would abstain from reconsidering her intention to perform some action once she settles on that action, unless her circumstances or information changes (Morton 2010, 563). In situations of scarcity and abundance, the Stability Norm makes sense so that the person can achieve ends of survival (in scarcity) or of living well (in abundance) without a disposition to change her mind about what really matters and what she needs given the situation. Morton notes that it is not always reasonable to hold to the Stability Norm: appropriate norms for deliberation and practical reasoning depend on the environment and the needs of the agent and other agents, her accountability to herself and others, and other considerations. Thus, even when guiding norms are identified, they must be flexible enough to account for domain-specificity.

Nevertheless, any account of domain-specificity in practical reasoning must be cautious not to unjustly exclude certain people from having ethical standing, being considerable, or taken as credible. When we deny the ethical standing of people, we restrict the scope of ethical principles in ways that marginalize and oppress some others. The question at hand is how to ground questions of who counts as considerable or credible without appeals to metaphysics and without staying stuck with particulars and local claims of ethical standing.

5.3.3 Intelligibility

Good enough practical reasoning requires that we be able to give reasons to others that explain why we did what we did and how we made sense of our behaviors and actions to ourselves. Sometimes, the norms that make sense to a person for himself or herself to act upon are different from the ones that others use in evaluating the agent's norms of deliberation (Morton 2010, 571). That explanation may be post hoc, but reasons-giving to others must be possible. Post hoc explanations are not the same as fabricated ones given merely to satisfy a questioner; they must, in some sense, be explanations that rest on beliefs, values, and perspectives that the explainer holds (whether tentatively or with conviction). Reasons-giving lends intelligibility to others of one's actions, where intelligibility means that others can follow those reasons. I suggest that the reasons given are adequate when they map onto a pattern of thought others can find themselves in if they apply themselves. (I discuss what it means for listeners to "apply themselves" in Chapter 6.) Sometimes a person's intensity of passion gets in the way of others' ability to view that person's actions as intelligible, and others' evaluations need to be cautious about not devaluing emotion—even intense emotion—because of its gendered and racialized associations. Still, sometimes even when one tries to understand another's reasons for behaving in such-and-such a way and one takes stereotypes and biases into consideration, one cannot make sense of the emotional intensity because it is objectively extreme and out-of-place. I say more about objectivity in Section 5.5.

Paul, in Chapter 4, explains why he hit Sam, in terms of feeling rejected by boys he wants to befriend him; after repeated rejections and the provocation that Sam whispers insults in Paul's ear, Paul hits Sam. The explanation regarding the provocation, plus Paul's decreasing ability to endure rejections by his peers, lends Paul's actions intelligibility. Nevertheless, Paul's reasons, though intelligible, are not acceptable, a point that I make clear in Section 5.3.5 on "accountability." Thus, intelligible practical reasoning is not the same as morally acceptable practical reasoning.

Another difficulty with the intelligibility feature is that those others to whom a person gives reasons may not consider the speaker to be credible. Consider Henry, whose psychiatrists diagnosed him with schizophrenia (Chapter 2). Henry rejects their diagnosis and treatments, putting himself at risk. His explanations—that he thinks his thinking is magical and enjoys it—is not counted as a good enough reason for psychiatrists to discharge him from hospital or discontinue anti-psychotics medications. Henry's ability to satisfy the reasons-giving feature of good practical reasoning prima facie is a reason for others to question his competence. Yet it is also important to ask ourselves who should count as the arbiter of what are considered to be "good reasons." I return to this point in Section 5.5.2.

Some readers might think that an intelligibility feature raises a problem regarding what should count as adequate sources of our reasons. Tessman, for example, offers an account of moral requirements that draws on intuitive as well as rational cognitive systems (see Box 5.2). Tessman employs both intuition and reason to explain how representation, affect, and behavioral aspects of cognitive processes give rise to moral requirement (Tessman 2015, see esp. ch. 2). This seems to present a challenge to my account of practical reasoning in that mine may seem to discount the role of intuition. I think Tessman's and my accounts are consistent, except that I am less comfortable with thinking of intuition and affect as a separate system from reason (current research notwithstanding).

5.3.4 **Followability**

In our world (meaning, the non-ideal global and interconnected world we live in today), we need a conception of practical reasoning that starts from the gritty realities of everyday life and that provides reasons for others to follow. It is not enough that reasons are convincing only within a limited domain, such as the reasons Paul gives for his physically aggressive behavior toward his

---

Box 5.2 Dual process theory

Current research in cognition suggests that at least some of our judgments are intuitive. Jonathan Haidt, for example, describes what is referred to in cognitive psychology as Dual Process Theory (DPT). Dual process theorists argue that two systems operate in cognitive processing: the intuitive system and the reasoning system (Croskerry 2009; Haidt 2001; Pelaccia et al. 2011). According to Haidt, the intuitive process is inaccessible and, although one can give post hoc reconstructions, one forges post hoc explanations out of results of actions, not out of the process itself (Haidt 2001). Applied to the clinician, the claim is that the intuitive system grasps the contextual and affective characteristics of a clinical encounter and is characterized by deliberation without attention, quick pattern recognition, and heuristics. Its advantages are that it is fast, natural, relatively effortless, and, it is claimed, more accurate (Croskerry 2009; Haidt 2001; see also Gladwell 2007). The other system, analytic, is characterized by abstract, decontextualized bounded rationality; it more closely approximates normative rationality and is robust. According to Haidt, the intuitive process is inaccessible and, although one can give post hoc reconstructions, one forges post hoc explanations out of results of actions, not out of the process itself (Haidt 2001).

peers. Paul's reasons are convincing in the sense that they provide an understanding to others as to why he hits and why he thinks it is a reasonable thing to do. But practical reasoning does not count as good reasoning if it is purely subjective and internal; since morality is social, moral reasons must be held intersubjectively. When we give reasons as to why we did or did not do something, we present those reasons as ones that others who fall within a given domain should also follow (O'Neill 1996, 58). Henry, who has schizophrenia, behaves in ways that are defiant but his behavior, at least for some actions, is not followable. That is, at least some of his behavior, such as his apparently complete disregard for actions that threaten his own life, cannot reasonably be presented as norms that others should follow.

I consider the following example to be an action that good practical reasoning would forbid us from adopting as a moral rule or norm. In early 2015, the Islamic State burned alive the Jordanian fighter pilot, First Lt. Moaz al-Kasasbeh. He had been captured and held in a cage after his plane was shot down. Images of the caged, burning body were then released as a video and quickly went viral. It is clear that burning someone alive is not an action that is followable in the sense either of "morally obligatory" or "permissible": moral beings would not wish such a death on anyone, let alone expect it to be a moral norm for others to follow—even within a restricted domain such as "members of the Islamic State." Actions that are intrinsically harmful are not followable even within a narrow domain (see Section 5.3.7 on harming).

Now consider hitting one's peers (Section 5.3.3 and 4.1). Parents and caregivers may teach parents a "principle of retaliation" that holds that, when another child hits you, you should hit back. That principle arguably is "followable" within a relevant domain; it also gives children who follow it a degree of intelligibility about their aggressive behaviors. Yet there is more to good enough practical reasoning than such a principle allows. Intelligibility and followability are important features of practical reasoning. Within cultures that hold such a principle or norm, people who are hit are accountable to hit back. However, such a principle may not entail a broader sense of accountability to others.

5.3.5 **Accountability**

Intelligibility provides understanding of others' behavior, attitudes, and actions, but often it does not legitimate behavior. Followability provides reasons for others to do what I do, but often those reasons are within a limited moral domain. One quality of good practical reasoning is that when we act, we understand ourselves to be doing so in the context of the social world(s) in which we live (whether particular or abstract). Margaret Walker frames morality as practices of responsibility that reveal what people value by making people accountable to those values (Walker 2007, 10). Practices of responsibility view people as answerable to one another; we answer to one another through discourses of accountability that include accepting or refusing, negotiating, excusing, showing regret, contempt, or indignation, apologizing, and making reparations (Walker 2007, 100). Being answerable and accountable to one another requires that we have the capacity and standing to speak for ourselves about ourselves, and to stand before others with the entitlement that we can and will place the same expectations on others (Walker 2007, 231). Tessman frames these ideas in terms of moral requirements. These requirements concern a plurality of moral values that indicate what actions are "called for"—or, I would add, call upon us to avoid, or prevent others from, doing (Tessman 2015). Answerability and accountability, thus, are mediated by obligations to respond to particular others, especially when those particular others are dependent on us (Walker 2007, 113). Most people experience themselves as having self-regarding moral requirements as well, and one of these may be to act defiantly in the face of unjust or oppressive circumstances.

Being accountable is one way that people can show others that they are trustworthy. Annette Baier says that "some degree of trust in the social world is the starting point and very basis of morality" (Baier 2004,180). I have argued that showing signs of one's trustworthiness is the responsibility especially of people who are in role-positions of authority or power, or who are advantaged by virtue of unequal social structures (Potter 2002). Some people cannot, and should not, take trust in others for granted. Given structural inequalities and the patterns of disadvantage and marginalization that are meted out, it sometimes is unwise to place trust in people in authority or who are in positions of power with respect to us, unless they have indicated their trustworthiness. The point is that, whether in distrusting others or otherwise responding to those in authority, we are accountable to ourselves as well as to others and, as I said in Chapter 4, sometimes people have self-regarding reasons to be defiant and to resist the pull to be held accountable to authoritative others. In an ideal world where individuals have full ethical standing, people are answerable and accountable to one another because they stand in reciprocal moral and legal relations. But in our world, where the majority of individuals are not accorded full ethical standing, answerability and accountability are usually asymmetrical (see Walker 2007, 215). Furthermore, to the extent that a person or patient cannot help what she or he does, that person's answerability and accountability are diminished. (For analyses of what it means to say that how one behaves is outside one's control, see Potter 2009; Mele 2005; Gert and Duggan 1979).

In the clinical domain, and with respect to patient defiance, these points raise pressing concerns. Most psychiatrists are deeply committed to practices that provide good care for their patients and, as good psychiatrists, they will acknowledge that they are accountable to patients, their families, the institutions in which they work, and the field of psychiatry itself. They recognize the asymmetry of clinician/patient relations. Furthermore, they often use their expertise and position of power to help patients and not to exercise undue authority and power over them. Yet psychiatrists may nevertheless overlook their patients' endeavors in practical reasoning that would justify defiant behaviors. They may inadvertently not grant as credible the reasoning processes of patients when they are defiant. Because the issues of accountability and voice are so complex, I reserve a discussion of them until Chapter 6.

5.3.6 **Spontaneity**

Aristotle's account of deliberation seems to suggest that it always is slow and proceeds cautiously. Good deliberation takes "a long time, and it is said that we must act quickly on the result of our deliberation, but deliberate slowly" (NE 1142b1–7). A slow procedural approach to deciding how to behave is meant to rule out good guessing about what is good to do, as well as to rule out impetuousity or what, in clinical circles, is called impulsivity. Guessing and impulsivity do not involve reasoning and are done quickly. Guessing toward good actions and behavior is unreliable because it is just as likely to lead us to bad as to good actions when we only try our luck at getting it right ethically. The impetuous or impulsive person is led by feelings (or by neuronal pathways, depending on the level of explanation). The good practical reasoner, if he notices something in advance, is not overcome by feelings but will be able to prepare himself through deliberation about the best course of action (1150b20–25). However, Aristotle allows that, in emergencies, we may act from a dispositional state without the usual "preparation" (NE 1117a17–22).

I take a critical stance on these strands of thinking. One feature of practical reasoning is that we pay attention to the people and problems that have standing within the relevant domain. I explained in Chapter 2 that acting from character requires background moral and intellectual development through habituation to seek what is good and fine and through training in prudence (practical reasoning). With good moral education in our childhoods, or with learning more about ourselves and the world as we mature, we learn to attend to and focus on salient moral issues and to overcome our own ignorance (leaving open what counts as salient, as that is locally shaped and not specified a priori). As Iris Murdoch says,

> if we consider what the work of attention is like, how continuously it goes on, and how imperceptibly it builds up structures of value round about us, we shall not be surprised that at crucial moments of choice most of the business of choosing

is already over . . . *What happens in between such choices is indeed what is crucial.* (Murdoch 1970, 37; emphasis added)

We do not need to rule out defiant behavior that seems to arise "out of nowhere." Instead, we need to know the background conditions that would give rise to defiance and understand how the defiant person reasoned toward her or his behavior. Additionally, as I have argued elsewhere, spontaneity itself is a worthwhile character trait. Of course, a distinction needs to be drawn between spontaneity and impulsivity, and often the difference seems to reside in outcomes: positive outcomes are praised as spontaneous while negative outcomes are regarded as indications of impulsivity (cf. Potter 2009). Spontaneity has an element of surprise, of breaking out of predictable patterns, and so being spontaneous involves taking risks. Yet spontaneous behavior may be guided by a larger conception of what makes that person's life worth living. The creativity and freedom experienced through spontaneity may be constitutive of living a good life. Nevertheless, being spontaneous requires a degree of self-monitoring even in creative acts. The background dispositions, the self-monitoring, and the expression of what makes life worth living lend credibility to a person's practical reasoning even when that reasoning does not include slow and deliberate thinking about what she or he should do. I especially want to highlight the relationship between spontaneity and passion. The priority given to reason over emotion and passion in most Western thought—David Hume (1975) is one notable exception, and Tessman (2015) is another—can lead people to accept the idea of the good rational person as one whose slow and deliberate practical reasoning keeps passion in its proper place and is moved to action by reason alone. In being defiant, however, passion frequently is an important positive quality of response and, the more it is tamped down and suppressed, the less likely it is to have the spark and energy that marks it off from mere disagreement, opposition, stubbornness, and other responses to authority. Of course, it matters what sorts of passion are brought to bear: homicidal rage is not a positive quality and so is not praiseworthy in any circumstances. The point is that spontaneity and passion go hand-in-hand, and this coupling does not mean that spontaneous responses devolve into impulsivity.

I have argued that norms of practical reasoning are important factors in evaluating defiant behavior both from the subjective experience of the person who is defiant and from the perspective of others. In reasoning about what to do or not do, one must also weight the risks and benefits of a particular course of action. This is not to say that all reasoning is consequentialist, but, instead, that part of reasoning about defiance will include weighing consequences— in particular, when it comes to comparative harms. Yet, as I will show in

Section 5.3.7, some harms are intrinsically wrong and ought never to be done or allowed. The question at hand is under what conditions one is justified in violating moral, social, and legal norms. To address these issues, I examine the concept of harms.

5.3.7 Harms

Reasoning well enough about behavior and actions most often will include the need for one to consider various harms both to others and to oneself. What gets counted as "harm" matters not only when we try to evaluate and address aggression, psychopathy, and clinically harmful behaviors, but also to the way a justice system functions. Philosophical literature on harms distinguishes between moral and non-moral harm, and between comparative and non-comparative harm (Peterson 2014). My position is that some harms are non-comparative, by which I mean that some harms are intrinsically bad, while other harms are comparative. Both concepts are relevant to practical reasoning. After I set out this distinction, I identify two ways that harms can be evaluated: intolerable harms and structurally produced vulnerability to harm. Although I discuss them separately, these two kinds of harm are interconnected and, as I will argue, they can provide justification for defiant behavior.

Thomas Peterson offers a theory of harm that he characterizes as morally neutral and comparative (Peterson 2014). Comparative harms are bad compared to some baseline, while non-comparative harms are bad states that are intrinsically bad. Peterson rejects a comparative concept of harms that requires an idea of baseline well-being and, instead, favors a counterfactual approach.[7] In his version of baseline comparative harms, one person is harmed by another if and only if by doing or allowing some act, that person brings it about that the other's level of well-being is lower than the well-being for humankind (Peterson 2014). His objection to this account of harms seems to be that it is not clear what that baseline would be or how to weigh differing harms. I think it is possible to address this objection, however.

Shlomit Harrosh defines harm relative to a humankind baseline of being able to engage with a basic human good, where to fully engage means "experiencing, finding meaning and value, setting ends, participation in activities and maintaining/being in certain states" with respect to a basic human good (Harrosh 2011, 4) It might be that such goods count as objective to the extent that people can construct a eudaimonistic human life by which to compare acts that impede their ability to engage with what makes life meaningful and worthwhile in this world. Still, I need to provide some context to the idea of basic harms and basic human goods. I draw on two philosophers to unpack these ideas: Claudia Card and Martha Nussbaum.

The starting point for Card in analyzing harms, evils, and atrocities is the concept of a tolerable life. She proposes that "a tolerable life is at least minimally worth living for its own sake and from the standpoint of the being whose life it is, not just as a means to the ends of others" (Card 2005,16). To understand the minimal requirements to make a life worth living, readers need a notion of basic harms. Basic harms are those that cause suffering through culpable wrongdoing. Basic harms are ones that no one should be made to endure. They include:

> such things as severe and unremitting pain; lacking access to unpolluted water, food, and air; severe and prolonged restrictions on motility (as in being confined to a box that allows one room neither to stand, sit, nor lie down); extreme and prolonged isolation; extreme and prolonged impotence or insecurity; and deprivation of the bases of self-respect and human dignity (including death with dignity). (Card 2002, 63)

Harms are not all equal; they are dimensional and come in a variety of unquantifiable degrees of severity, such as intensity of suffering and the effects on one's ability to function (Card 2002, 14). Intolerable harms coupled with culpable wrongdoing produce evils, according to Card (although this is not an area that I address). I believe that being oppressed should be considered to be an intolerable harm: it undermines the basis of self-respect and dignity. For many people, oppression is an enduring condition of material and psychological insecurity and instability; racism, sexism, and gender normativity are intolerable harms in this sense (see Chapter 4). It might be the case that the ability of people living with a mental illness to experience themselves as self-respecting people who sometimes are credible, or who are credible about some things, is undermined by their encounters in psychiatry. To the extent that this is an ongoing experience or produces an enduring state of self-denigration, self-distrust, and self-doubt, it might be considered an intolerable harm. While I might be stretching Card's idea of intolerable harm beyond her position, I press the point that the relationship between people with mental illnesses, or who are at risk of being evaluated as having mental illnesses, may experience intolerable harms. Such experiences may justify defiant behavior.

Card offers a description of basic harms; Nussbaum, as I discussed in Chapter 3, gives an account of basic goods known as "capabilities." The ten capabilities she identifies are: life; bodily health; bodily integrity; senses, imagination, and thought; emotions; practical reason; affiliation; living with concern for other species; play; and control over one's environment (see Box 3.2). Nussbaum claims that these capabilities are universal and capture something essential in what it means to be able to live a life worthy of human dignity. I am less sure of a universal claim to essential capabilities than I am of a description of intolerable harms; there is an intuitive sense to Card's discussion of intolerable harms and is more difficult to grasp when it comes to claims about basic goods. The identification of what "human beings" need is such an encompassing conceptual task that it can seem epistemically challenging to make claims in this regard and not import privileged Western values. But I think we can use Nussbaum's idea to think about what constitutes egregious harms. Egregious harms are ones that prevent people, or groups of people, from exploring or realizing some of the characteristics or qualities that make life worth living.

Intolerable harms are intrinsically bad, as are denials of basic capabilities. They would be, in Peterson's theory, non-comparable harms. Still, not all harms are intrinsic and non-comparable. To explain this point, I turn to Joel Feinberg. Feinberg distinguishes between a harmful condition and a harmed one. A harmful condition is one that has adverse effects on that person's overall well-being; an example of this might be severe mental illness. A harmed condition is a harmful condition that is the result of harming (Feinberg 1990, 26). Both kinds of harm are important in thinking about patients who are defiant, because patients interface with the institution of psychiatry, and psychiatry has a history of being oppressive (Chapter 2, Section 2.3.2). So, even those in harmful conditions due to mental illness may be harmed by psychiatry, and the question then is when it would be reasonable for some patients to behave defiantly as a response to being harmed. Some acts of harming are intrinsically bad—such as oppressing other persons or groups of people—and, at the same time, they are comparative. It is important to remember that oppression is a harmful condition of being structurally and unjustifiably burdened at the expense of some other group or groups that structurally and unjustifiably benefit from actions and practices that oppress.

One way to understand when defiance is harmful to others is in terms of structural vulnerabilities or risks of vulnerabilities. Feinberg sets out necessary and sufficient conditions for one person to have harmed another (Feinberg 1990, 26). He frames acts of harming in terms of interests and rights, a view that entails a conception of individuals as rights-bearers who have competing interests. While I believe that an individualist conception of the person is mistaken, I think the concerns about vulnerability have merit. My way of implementing Feinberg's theory of harming is to say that a person (or group or institution) harms another person (or group or institution) when that person's intentional or negligent acting creates vulnerability, risks of vulnerability, or other adverse consequences to the other person, and that that person's acting is neither excusable nor justifiable and hence is indefensible. Some vulnerabilities, and thus some harmful conditions, are unavoidable, but other harmful conditions are humanly caused (either intentionally or negligently). And some of those humanly caused harmful conditions are unjustifiable. Some people are in a position to protect the vulnerable from (more) harms (Goodin 1985), and a moral requirement is placed on those people not to harm and to avoid harming. According to Tessman, the motivation to fulfill such a moral requirement arises out of our affective experience (Tessman 2015, 70). While I am less inclined than Tessman to favor a dichotomy between intuition and reason, I think the role of affect that she highlights is important not only in identifying moral requirements of not-harming but also in capturing the centrality of affect to being defiant when one is being harmed in ways that exacerbate structural vulnerabilities. Tessman and I are in agreement that affective and passionate character qualities should be acknowledged for their central place in ethical life and, I argue, in virtuous defiance in particular. Jesse Prinz's work is helpful here. Prinz argues that intuitions, in that they draw upon affect and feelings, can yield "oughtitudes"—affective attitudes that prescribe moral actions (Prinz 2007). We have emotional dispositions about particular actions—meaning whether or not we ought to do those actions, and whether or not others ought to have done particular actions—and it is these emotional dispositions that give rise to an affective "ought" or what Prinz calls a prescriptive sentiment (Prinz 2007). So, one feature of good defiance is that it arises from an oughtitude, one that will, in some circumstances, prescribe defiant behavior that does not contribute to intolerable harms or that, at least, does not cause or contribute to greater unjust and oppressive harms, or vulnerabilities to harms, than ordinary actions do (see Section 5.3).

5.4 **Contestability**

Prevailing accounts of reason assume not only that norms of reasonableness (that is, norms that require identifying the necessary means to reach an action-end, consistency in being moved for the right reasons and toward the right end, and so on) guide practical deliberation, but that there is only one set of those norms. I have argued that, in order for our actions to count as reasonable ones to perform, we need to be able to give reasons for choosing a particular action. Giving reasons, though, turns out to require that those reasons follow certain norms for justification. Many believe that people who respond to those norms in appropriate ways are reasonable. I am inclined to think that people who engage in practical reasoning such as I have sketched so far do indicate reasonableness. But, because the stakes are so high when the line between reason/unreason or functional/dysfunctional is drawn, I also believe that readers need to be wary of pronouncements on what counts as reasonable. It matters greatly what people mean by those norms of reasonableness, where they come from, and who decides that a particular set of norms is best. Critics are rightly concerned that most accounts of practical reasoning are reified and inflexible. Amélie Rorty challenges philosophers who persist in looking for the foundational norms for deliberation and practical reasoning: "for better or worse, the process of formulating the criteria for rationality—its basic aims, structures, and norms—is itself open to the multiperspectival, critical reevaluation" (Rorty 2004, 280).[8]

The idea of reasoning well, what counts as reasons, and who decides such matters is linked with some of the concerns of epistemology. I have in mind issues of who counts as knowers, what it means to be epistemically responsible, and how situations of epistemic injustice occur. I delve into these issues in Chapter 6; here, I argue that a central part of being epistemically and morally responsible is to be willing to engage critically with claims about practical reasoning. I unpack this idea in terms of a particular way of understanding objectivity known as "strong objectivity."

According to Donna Haraway, the task of scientists (and, specifically, for readers of this book, psychiatrists) is to simultaneously honor the historical contingency of knowledge claims and knowing subjects and hold fast to a commitment to accounts of a real metaphysical world (Haraway 1988, 579). Drawing on Haraway's work, I suggest a critical perspective on how meanings and knowers get made, not to deny their reality but to build meanings and knowing subjects that resonate with people's lived experiences and joys and sufferings (Haraway 1988, 580). Haraway argues that we can create objectivity only through partial perspectives because situated knowledge entails embodiment, which has limited location. Embodied knowledge differs from unlocatable knowledge claims because the latter cannot be called to account. This does not commit her—or me—to relativism, however:

> The alternative to relativism is not totalization and single vision, which is always finally the unmarked category whose power depends on systematic narrowing and obscuring. The alternative to relativism is partial, locatable, critical knowledge sustaining the possibility of webs of connections called solidarity in politics and shared conversations in epistemology. (Haraway 1988, 584)

I take seriously Haraway's idea of a practice of objectivity that privileges contestation while honoring and trusting in local, situated knowledges. "Location," she says, "resists the politics of closure" (Haraway 1988, 590). She uses the metaphor of vision to suggest that the object of knowledge be pictured as an actor, a subject, and not a passive thing or object, a knower in his or her own right. Psychiatry, then, is not so much a practice of discovery but of conversation.

Lorraine Code frames epistemic normativity in terms of ecological thinking, which "offers a better "way of inhabiting the world"" and provides a "model of reciprocally informing and sustaining, critically interrogating practices of engaged inquiry" (Code 2006, 7, 90). The emphasis on ecology is significant in that it highlights the need to understand interdependent organisms in their habitat while developing strategies of knowing well that do not exploit either habitats or other inhabitants (Code 2006, 91). Any application of norms to particular people or patients, then—whether those norms are legal or non-legal, linguistic, moral, or social—requires that we attend to the particularities of local knowledge and local practices. Such understanding in turn requires that we learn "how to hear, interpret, and act upon evidence from testimonial sources not commonly accorded authoritative voice." (Code 2008, 38). Privileged and dominant knowers need to be critical of our own inclination and training to import our schemas, stereotypes, assumptions, and interpretations onto others. Local knowers, when granted credibility (for example, about what local illness is and how best to treat it [Code 2008]) often better serve the needs of various populations than an imposition of widely assumed "universal" methods and truths. I have argued that norms of reasoning need to be inclusive, by which I mean that local knowledge and subjective knowing needs to be able to expand from particular locales and situations in order not to be strictly relative. Still, local knowledge cannot merely be extended from one site to another; it needs to be tested. As Code explains, it must be capable "of withstanding serious epistemic and practical-political scrutiny" (Code 2008, 39). I take it that part of what Code means by the need to test local knowledge is that we need to learn, over time, not just which effects occur temporarily, or with regard to some event or occurrence (such as local responses of traditional healers to Ebola in a particular region of Sierra Leone in 2014), but what norms serve a particular group of people over time and why. It also includes that we do not merely assume that local knowledge is transferable to new locales. Learning what serves local populations best over time requires a particular epistemic stance.

That stance challenges some of the assumptions within science, including psychiatry. Conventional norms of objectivity require that knowledge be discovered through processes that eliminate bias and subjectivity. But, as this book has argued, what counts as subjective interests and values differs in different groups. The result is that assumptions may be invisible or may seem unquestionable to those inside a given scientific or psychiatric practice:

> Because of this "objectivity effect" [the fiction of objectivity] the membership of epistemic communities and the relations among their members become crucial. A sound epistemic practice has to look critically at the practices, relations, and background assumptions within its own community. (Walker 2007, 64–5)

One epistemological response to the view from nowhere is to claim that some group of people, in virtue of their marginalized or oppressed lived conditions—say, working-class people, or minority women, or victims of a genocidal regime—have a privileged viewpoint from which to see more clearly the reality of our everyday world. As I showed in Chapter 4 with respect to children's intersectionalities, however, local norms and knowledges are always situated within overlapping and broader contexts; there is no such thing as an entirely isolated and untouched group of knowers who exist somewhere in the world as we know it. Knowers, Sandra Harding (1993) says, are multiple, heterogeneous, and contradictory or incoherent, and we cannot rest knowledge on any one group's supposed privileged epistemic position. So, the idea that some class of people has a privileged epistemic standpoint cannot be justified because knowers must make sense of local knowledge and knowing in the context of other people in other groups whose lives invariably touch one other. What we need is a kind of objectivity that allows for ongoing critique, challenge, and negotiation.

Sandra Harding proposes the practice of "strong objectivity," by which she means that epistemic communities need to examine critically their own practices, interests, assumptions, and biases. They need to notice and, often, contest, the tools and measures and the attitudes toward their objects of study—in the case of psychiatry, the people or patients themselves (Harding 1993). Harding argues that the practice of objectivism "impoverishes its attempts at maximizing objectivity when it turns away from the task of critically identifying all of those broad, historical social desires, interests, and values that have shaped the agendas, contents, and results of the sciences much as they shape the rest of human affairs" (Harding 1993, 70). As Walker says, strong objectivity requires that people examine assumptions of cognitive authority in order to ensure that it does not disguise dominance or suppress criticism from diverse viewpoints (Walker 2007, 65).

O'Neill says that making ethical judgments involves affirming not only the way of life for "our" in-group, but also what could be judged for others as worthy activities, lives, and institutions (O'Neill 1996, 88). I will add that this requires that we adopt the stance of strong objectivity so that we do not simply import and impose privileged and advantaged conceptions of what makes a life worth living. We are accountable to others both known and unknown (unknown by omission but also by intention) to construct, and to leave open for others to construct, accounts of worthwhile living activities that allow for diverse and local world-views but that take seriously the suffering caused and harms done by disability, oppression, and burdened virtues.

I apply the idea of strong objectivity to norms of practical reasoning, especially as they pertain to assessments of the reasonableness of patients' defiant behavior. If psychiatry adopts norms of practical reasoning such as the ones I discuss in Section 5.3 and does not build into those norms the feature of contestability, it may create more moral damage than good and, as an institution, it runs the risk of being epistemically arrogant or unjust even if individual psychiatrists are well intentioned. In ethics as in science, knowers, actor/subjects, and evaluators need to employ strong objectivity. The conclusion of Section 5.4 is that members of epistemic communities in psychiatry need to take a critical stance on their status as experts and authoritative knowers about what counts as reasonable beliefs, dysfunctional states, traits that are biologically given, and, in the theme of this book, persistent defiance as a dysfunction instead of a potentially virtuous disposition.

I have presented features both of practical reasoning and of intolerable harms that frame defiant behavior more clearly as a virtue or a vice. The implication of this analysis is that some cases of defiance will be intelligible, followable, and otherwise justifiable. My theory of defiance as a virtue is now clearer. Defiance is a virtue when it:

a. arises out of a response to basic or egregious harms such as oppression or injustice
b. is self-preserving
c. expresses at least some components of practical reasoning
d. expresses a mean for affect and passion
e. is done from a dispositional state
f. does not contribute to harms that are themselves oppressive or unjust.

If a person's defiant behavior is to be considered good, that behavior needs to arise out of an ability to read or interpret situations and to feel the appropriate affective sense or passionate awareness that defiance is called for. The defiant person needs to draw on at least some of the norms of practical reasoning and to assess the harms and self-preserving benefits involved. Defiance may harm others and still be considered good, such as when the harm is to thwart the continued success of structural and unjust advantages. (Arguably, President Obama's executive order signing into law immigration reform is a move to decrease exploitation among illegal and migrant workers, while opposition cries "harm!" because it may take away opportunities for that very exploitation to occur through access to low-wage workers as well as opportunities to punish illegal entry into the United States.) Additionally, a person might either be defiant out of a characteristic state or be defiant as a particular response. Either can be good, but only the former is a virtue given the definition of a virtue. Finally, whether or not defiance is a virtue will vary in particular contexts and within given local ecologies (see Chapter 4, Section 4.6). Yet it can be objectively determined within the constraints of objectivity I have described.

In Section 5.5, I return to two cases (one from Chapter 3 and one from this chapter) to see what light is shed on defiant behavior when considering the features of practical reasoning presented in Section 5.3. and the contestability requirement in Section 5.4.

5.5 Reprise on two cases

5.5.1 Christian Gerhartsreiter

As I have explained, I reject merely subjective and relativist reasoning on both epistemic and ethical grounds. Yet I take seriously the subjective experience of those whose affective and dispositional sense is that they are being treated unjustly, discredited, pathologized, or further oppressed. Such experiences may lead people to behave defiantly, and it is my contention that many of them draw on features of practical reasoning to motivate their behavior.

However, as I discussed in Chapter 2, people may be defiant without having the experience of being oppressed or treated unfairly. Gerhartsreiter's actions are a case in point. He seemed to be guided by instrumental reasoning but, as I understand his story, he was not guided by features of practical reasoning such as those I identify. He is not inclusive in the sense described by Walker that moves one from subjective or local norms and values toward shared norms, principles and maxims; instead, his imposturing relies precisely on not holding shared norms. His actions may be intelligible to some others—he likely is able to give reasons for his actions—but those reasons themselves would be suspect because they are likely founded on deception. I say this because he cannot reveal his deceptions and still operate fraudulently. His actions are not followable, nor would any person who globally exempts himself from norms and expectations want them to be followable. Gerhartsreiter gets away with his defiance and deceptions only if others do not detect his motives and intentions, let alone apply them to themselves.

The feature of answerability is more complicated. Gerhartsreiter does not appear to consider himself to be accountable to anyone except himself, so he would seem to fail this characteristic of practical reasoning. Yet I argued in Chapter 4 that sometimes it is reasonable and even virtuous to answer to one-self and disregard the expectation that one's behavior be accountable to particular others. The difference is found in the discussion of harms that form the parameters of good defiance. Defensible defiance arises out of a response to basic harms; is self-preserving; expresses some components of practical reasoning; is done from a dispositional state; and does not contribute to harms that are themselves oppressive or unjust. As with others who fulfill the criteria for ASPD, Gerhartsreiter (although not publicly stated as having ASPD) performs actions that, over time, indicate an almost complete disregard for the concerns of others. I have argued elsewhere that lying and deception are not always wrong, but his behavior does not meet with justifiable exceptions to a general norm against calculating self-interested deceit (Potter 2002, ch. 2). While his arts of deception and imposturing are dispositional, he defies epistemic, legal, moral, and social norms for reasons that are unjustifiable. His global and long-standing defiance is wrong because it leaves others vulnerable to risks that they do not know about and are not undertaking through their own agency and, as far as I know, his imposturing was not prompted by experiences of structural vulnerabilities or oppressive conditions. In fact, Gerhartsreiter seems to lack the qualities that would make possible the oughtitudes for moral motivations (see Section 5.3.7). He and other people who exhibit characteristics of ASPD such as lack of empathy and other affective deficits may have disordered personality characteristics that inhibit or prevent them from engaging in the kind of practical reasoning I describe, in part because they cannot draw upon prescriptive sentiments that provide moral reasons for action. This way of understanding ASPD and psychopathology has been contested, however. John Deigh (2014), for example, drives a wedge between the capacity to feel moral emotions such as attachment and resentment and the capacity to reason morally. He argues that even the psychopathic killer may have the capacity for moral emotions but not the capacity to reason morally.[9] (See Schramme 2014 for a collection of essays on such questions.) The upshot, at any rate, is that the behavior of Gerhartsreiter, counts as bad defiance.

5.5.2 **Henry**

In Chapter 3, I considered whether Henry Cockburn's behavior could qualify as good or reasonable defiance. Henry, readers may recall, has been diagnosed with schizophrenia. He does not accept his diagnosis and interprets his unusual cognitive experiences as "magical." When he refuses medication, escapes from hospitals, and exposes himself to natural elements in ways that risk his life, he defies the concerns of psychiatrists and his family. I am now in a position to clarify how I would situate Henry's defiance. Henry's perspective, although subjective, needs to be taken seriously because the contestability feature of practical reasoning requires that assessments by others do not assume the correctness of prevailing norms for reason. It is difficult to see his behavior as intelligible or followable, but part of that difficulty may reside in evaluators' established epistemic commitments (including my own). That is, from within a given epistemic practice, such as psychiatry, it is a challenge to understand others whose world-view seems radically different—for example, in patients with schizophrenia. Yet it is possible and even necessary for psychiatrists to learn to understand the world of a patient who is mentally ill from that patient's perspective through what is called "world"-traveling, a concept I borrow from María Lugones (Potter 2003). World-traveling, in this context, is the willful exercise of shifting from one's more comfortable world of experience in a way that decenters oneself. It involves witnessing the patient as she sees and experiences herself, with her struggles, her values, and sometimes her epistemological idiosyncrasies. If psychiatrists do this traveling to patients' worlds, they may find that the behavior of many patients does have at least some degree of intelligibility. When we allow that the norms of practical reasoning are contestable, we may come to understand some behavior not as symptomatic of severe mental illness but as within the scope of defiance, and subject to praise or blame.

Yet, I cannot say that Henry's defiance should be praised. It nearly kills him and he does not seem to have good reasons to die—even from the perspective of strong, contestable objectivity. His actions, although intelligible (as I have argued), are mostly not followable. But I will say that it is *in the direction of* praiseworthy defiance. I am influenced by people who are living with mental illnesses and who frame both their mental illness and their encounters with psychiatry as things they need to recover from. These writers demand that their own perspectives and their developing goals should be central in learning to live with a mental illness and that they should not have their mental illnesses framed in terms of debilitating symptoms, suffering, and incapacitation. Fred Frese, Edward Knight, and Ellyn Saks, all of whom have been diagnosed with schizophrenia, write that many recovering people "characterized the [psychiatric] treatment they had experienced as oppression, often viewing professionals as part of the oppressive mental health system" (Frese, Knight, and Saks 2009, 371). They explain that the first tenet of recovery for service users is that of self-direction (Frese, Knight, and Saks 2009, 372).[10] Thinking about living with mental illness as a matter of recovery is a way of reframing it as a question of how to live well with its challenges. Given my account of flourishing (see Chapter 3), I might initially have said that Henry's defiance was unlikely to contribute to his living well. After all, advocating self-direction usually does not imply the extreme life-threatening actions that Henry took (although it is worth pointing out that those who engage in life-threatening extreme sports are self-directed yet typically are viewed as fairly reasonable). It also seems clear that, at the time the book *Henry's demons* was written, Henry was not yet prepared to think in terms of recovery. Still, the perspective of recovery provokes a shift in how to conceptualize Henry's behavior. Paradoxically, even though Henry put himself in situations that were deadly, he might also have been expressing a self-directed, appropriate instinct toward self-preservation. That is, he might rightly have feared psychiatry as a potentially oppressive force that deprived him of a sense of self-worth. I believe that Henry's psychiatrists were right to be concerned about his ability to assess situations and to evaluate potential self-harms and self-destruction. They were also concerned with the suffering that Henry's family were experiencing, something Henry himself seemed less sensitive to. In evaluating Henry's defiant behavior, psychiatrists and others need to take into account a complicated assessment of Henry's reasoning and actions that makes a central place for Henry's point of view and that opens up the lens from which his behavior can be considered to be in the direction of praiseworthy defiance.[11]

In the final chapter of this book, I focus on the sorts of things that psychiatrists can do to respond appropriately and helpfully to patients' defiance. I frame the argument in that chapter in terms of epistemological and ethical responsibilities, addressing two virtues that psychiatrists can cultivate in this context: what I call "giving uptake" and what I recommend as psychiatrists' own brand of being defiant.

Chapter 6

The virtue of giving uptake in psychiatry

In this chapter, I address the question of what psychiatrists can and should do with the analysis presented in this book. I consider questions of what it means to see and be seen, to listen and be listened to, to know and be known, and how we learn our ways of seeing, listening, and knowing. Additionally, I ask why well-meaning, even enlightened, people fail to see that their ways of seeing, of treating and of constructing other persons as Other (see Introduction) can undermine the best of intentions and sometimes do harm. Chapter 6 addresses those questions by bringing together ethical and epistemological issues that provide some direction in responding to patients' and other people's defiant behavior. First, I introduce the virtue of giving uptake properly, and I argue that psychiatrists should cultivate a disposition to give uptake to defiant patients. This virtue is not the only one that can be useful in responding to defiance—empathy, trustworthiness, and *phronesis* are some others—but giving uptake is especially valuable and, since it is rarely discussed, it is important for psychiatrists to know about. Giving uptake is not easy to do well, though, and in Section 6.2, I consider epistemic impediments to giving uptake properly. First, I place broader social practices of ignorance and needing not to know under scrutiny by introducing theories called epistemologies of ignorance and epistemologies of resistance. In Section 6.3, after explaining what philosophers mean by these ideas, I say how they might apply to psychiatry. I argue that the kind of problems in psychiatric practice that I identify can affect psychiatrists' disposition to give uptake well and, in particular, to people who behave defiantly. In Section 6.4, I will work through a case to illustrate these impediments. Section 6.5 offers a hypothetical case that indicates how giving uptake to a defiant patient would look in a more idealized version. I conclude by drawing together some threads of the book.

6.1 The virtue of giving uptake

I have argued that defiance, under some circumstances, is an appropriate response to oppressive norms and living with adverse conditions. An appropriate response exists to defiance, as well, and it is to interact with a defiant person in a way that does not exacerbate that person's distress or struggles. As Tessman argues (2005, ch. 3), those who are in positions of significant power and authority, whether role authority and/or the authority of political, social, and economic power, need to work on their character as well. That is, people in positions of authority and power, as psychiatrists are, ought to actively avoid domination and work to change abusive and unjust structures and disciplines. One way to do so is to cultivate virtues that are responsive to attempts to assert one's worth, to maintain one's dignity, or to challenge the status quo, by being defiant. I will focus on one virtue.[1]

6.1.1 **Background of the concept of uptake**

Uptake is a term introduced by J.L. Austin, who argues that when we use words, we are doing much more than merely passively representing an already existing fact—we are performing actions and bringing new facts into existence (Austin 1975). Speech acts, therefore, are a subset of actions. Austin suggests that philosophers have paid more attention to the content of an utterance (what is called the locutionary act) and the effects of an utterance (the perlocutionary act), but have tended to overlook the action that is constituted by the utterance itself (the illocutionary act). For example, when I say, "the cat is on the mat," one might think that this saying (the locutionary act) is just a report of what is already true, but Austin says that the performative aspect of it brings the cat and the mat, as well as the location of the cat, into existence. Some actions, such as warning and promising, are illocutionary, and certain illocutionary acts have to produce certain effects on the listener in order to count as successful (Austin 1975). The successful performance of some illocutionary acts is what Austin calls uptake—that is, securement by the listener of the illocutionary act performed (see Figure 6.1).

Austin argues that uptake is a speech convention that is necessary in order for certain speech acts to come off. As I say, only certain illocutionary acts require that the listener gives uptake to the speaker. Speech acts such as warning, military ordering, or calling "out," do not require it, even though they

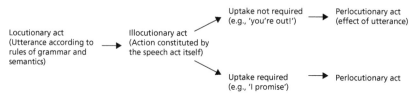

Fig. 6.1 Sketch of Austin's theory of speech acts.

are illocutionary—meaning that they perform acts themselves (i.e., they are performative). For example, when a judge warns a lawyer that, if he interrupts again, he will be held in contempt of court, that warning may not have the desired perlocutionary effect of silencing the lawyer, but the actual perform-ance of the act—the warning—is not dependent on the listener recognizing or acknowledging that a particular illocutionary act has been performed. Or suppose a tornado is approaching but you didn't receive any warning. If the weather service posted a warning, then even if you didn't hear about it, the warning still occurred. The reason, in this case, is that a weather service warn-ing has an institutionalized performance and its illocutionary act is labeled "WARNING." So, the occurrence of the action is separable from the produc-tion of its desired effect. Similarly, when an umpire calls "out," that fact is brought into existence regardless of whether or not the listeners acknowledge the "out" as a fact. Warning, calling "out," or ordering are illocutionary acts that do not require securement.

Other illocutionary acts, such as promising, apologizing, and betting, do require securing uptake from the listener. For example, one cannot be said to have made a promise if the listener does not recognize it as a promise. When a person gives uptake to his partner's words of "I do" or "I will" in a wedding ceremony, that listener is acknowledging that the speaker has placed himself under a specific set of obligations (such as making a commitment to be sup-portive to his partner). In order to give uptake, the listener must demonstrate acknowledgment through some kind of response. In wedding ceremonies where promises are articulated in speech acts, the promise-making might be followed by a kiss, a heartfelt embrace, or a wedding knot. Another example is that of promising to keep a confidence. Suppose Tim tells Marguerite that he is having an affair and asks her not to tell his partner Peter. Did she make a promise? According to Austin's theory, she only promised if two things occur: she performs a speech act of promising, and Tim gives her uptake on that promise. (Therefore, Marguerite might deny that she promised confiden-tiality when she agreed to keep the affair secret; she tells Tim that she never technically promised. I'll return to promising shortly.) Or, suppose I say to Ahmed "What do you want to bet that Sally will be late again?" and he replies "How about lunch?" Then, when Sally is late and I want Ahmed to pay for lunch, if he exclaims "We never made a bet!" what has mis-fired? Ahmed is claiming that the bet did not "come off" because he did not formally agree to it. That is, betting requires acknowledgment from the listener that the speaker has made a bet, and that acknowledgment would entail securement through a handshake or by saying, "It's a deal" or some other formalized response. In sum, promising, betting, and apologizing call for the active response of the listener in order to "seal" the meaning of those speech acts, and that active response is called "uptake."

Austin's theory of speech acts offers a useful insight into the importance of actively securing meaning between people, and he points to a broader, and much more complicated, concern about how to determine successful or unsuccessful communications. As my examples will suggest, clear cases are almost never found unless there is an institutionalized formal ritual, and many ambiguous cases can be disambiguated non-linguistically—as in looking a person in the eye, shaking another's hand—or dialogically. While I am attracted to Austin's idea about uptake, I will briefly point out three shortcomings.[2] First, it is too thin a conception of securing meaning: it applies only to certain performative utterances such as promising, and it requires only that the listener acknowledge superficially that those utterances were performed; second, it is too restricted in that it assumes relative equals in its theory; and third, it is too narrow in that the domain of uptake is only that of words. I expand upon Austin's notion of uptake while still retaining the need for meaning to be secured between parties.

Regarding the first concern, I question Austin's conception of uptake such that it occurs as long as acknowledgment has been given. I agree that, without the acknowledgment that a speech act has occurred, uptake will not be secured (Potter 2002). However, a question arises as to whether or not to count a speech act as having been given uptake when the listener acknowledges that an illocutionary act has occurred but does not accept the locution in its deeper intended meaning. For example, Lucy has failed to keep her commitment to be a good friend to Daniela. Lucy might passionately say "I am going to do better!" but Daniela does not believe her. She might not doubt her intentions, but does doubt her ability to follow through over time. She might be aware that Lucy faces what Tessman calls "impossible moral demands"—demands that encumber virtue in Lucy's lived conditions (Tessman 2015). Daniela might be said to acknowledge that the friend makes a promise, but she does not allow that promise to get a toe-hold. In my view, Daniela has not given uptake to Lucy even though she understands Lucy to be placing herself under a binding oath. Furthermore, when she withholds uptake, then Daniela cannot later say that Lucy broke her promise if Lucy fails to follow through, but she can say this if she does give uptake to Lucy's promising and Lucy does not follow through. The United States National Security Agency might receive threats from Al Qaeda that it refuses to be alarmed by. It recognizes that a threat is made but doesn't allow those threats to get a toe-hold. Even ordering is complicated. A soldier might acknowledge that an order has been given but refuses to follow it, in which case it looks like the solider has given uptake. Yet one might be ordered to do something and refuse to recognize the order *as an order* because one does not recognize the orderer's authority over oneself. Or consider an individual making a request to her manager. If a migrant worker says, "I want work!" and then is hired, but the manager requires her to work 16-hour days in order to keep her position as a worker, her intended meaning of "work" cannot be said to have been given uptake. The manager acknowledges that the worker made a request and he responds to that request, but the work requirements given were not what the worker meant by her request. The manager exploits the ambiguity of the word "work" by deliberately violating context-dependent linguistic norms.

In each of these cases of promising, threatening, ordering, and requesting, the listener acknowledges that an illocutionary act has occurred, but his or her refusal to interpret the speech act as carrying the deeper meaning that the speaker intends leaves open the question of whether uptake has occurred. I would argue that it has not. Additionally, as the example of requests shows, the kind of response one gives is crucial to giving uptake properly. That is, giving uptake places constraints on what counts as appropriate responses to another's communicative act. Austin seems to think that, as long as the listener receives the speech act as having a certain meaning, that speech act is secured. This is a thin sense of giving uptake, however. Of course, listeners do not always (as my examples might imply) intentionally or consciously acknowledge a speech act but not its intended meaning, but this only points to the great challenge that giving uptake well presents—and the reason I focus on uptake and its impediments in this chapter.

The second shortcoming in Austin's ideas about uptake is that he seems only to consider it as an occurrence between equals. According to Austin, giving uptake is an act that the listener performs in order to affirm that he or she has grasped the speaker's meaning of her illocutionary act. But Austin confines his analysis to what he takes to be the conventional meaning of speech acts, such as promising or warning. His analysis thus rests on the assumption of shared conventional meanings—assumptions that neither the advantaged nor the disadvantaged in hegemonic societies seem to hold. I have argued that it frequently is more difficult for people who are disadvantaged or subordinated, or who live under adverse conditions—for instance, Henry, from Chapter 3, who has been diagnosed with schizophrenia and lives with a mental disorder as well as the stigma that attaches to it—to secure uptake from people with more advantages (see Potter 2000). One central problem in stratified societies is that people who live under adverse conditions, or whose lives are structured by oppression, are not taken to be credible, or as credible as those with greater authority. Thus, their communicative acts are discounted, distorted, or even ignored—that is, not counted as speech acts. In the latter case, it is as if one has not spoken at all (see Potter 2000). Epistemologies of ignorance or resistance might be at play here, and one way the epistemological issues show up is in the ways that uptake is more or less likely to be given depending on the social position one is in. I return to this point in Section 6.3. Another problem is that disadvantaged people may be considered a threat to the status quo—to conventions and norms and civil society—and thus taken to pose some danger. It's not that they are not taken to be credible, but that they are taken to be untrustworthy with respect to the maintenance of social structures. In this case, the communicator might indeed mean to disable or fracture the authority of another person or institutional structure.

The third shortcoming of Austin's notion of uptake is that it frames uptake entirely in terms of speech acts. I frame it more broadly: giving uptake is a communicative act with ethical dimensions. As such, it is not restricted to speech acts (let alone only certain speech acts). We communicate through sighs, the tone and energy with which we speak, the look in our eyes, our body language, the length of time it takes us to respond to another, and so on. We can communicate through silence, as Adrienne Rich writes:

> Silence can be a plan
> rigorously executed
>
> the blueprint to a life
>
> It is a presence
> it has a history   a form
>
> Do not confuse it
> with any kind of absence (Rich 1978, 17)

This broader theory of uptake, as I have developed it, involves a particular kind of communicating. It reorients the listener to the speaker as a subject whose communications are worthy of consideration. Admittedly, to conceive of uptake in this broader way is a departure from Austin's original idea, and I am not the first person to notice his use of the concept of "uptake" and to broaden it. Marilyn Frye said of women's anger that it is not given uptake but, instead, is trivialized, mocked, pathologized, and ignored. "Deprived of uptake, the woman's anger is left as just a burst of expression of individual feeling. As a social act, an act of communication, it just doesn't happen" (Frye 1983, 89). Frye does not develop a theory of uptake, as I do, but she captures what I believe is Austin's important insight into the securing of meaning between people.

Everyday English usage of the term suggests that we do take the concept of "uptake" to carry this broader meeting. For example, suppose your friend has gone to a difficult meeting in which she requests funding from the Arts Council and, upon returning, exclaims to you, "I didn't get any uptake whatsoever!" Or, during an intense and conflictual conversation between spouses, one might say to the other, "Come on, I need some uptake here." Even in Spanish or French, the idea of uptake seems to be at play in ordinary language. For example, in Spanish street vernacular, "uptake" typically means "comprender/comprensión/entendimiento." But it sometimes is related to credibility. Consider the usage from English to Spanish: "The police didn't investigate because they didn't give him any uptake" to "La policía no investigó/no llevó a cabo una investigación porque no le creyó/porque él no le pareció creíble/porque él no era creíble/por su falta de credibilidad/etc."[3] A French version of "uptake" would be the translation of "He did not take the request/comment into consideration." This reflects that the person had a choice and opted not to take the speaker seriously.[4]

6.1.2 Giving uptake as a virtue

I define uptake as dialogical responsiveness and openness in the context of plurality and systemically stratified society. It involves respecting, attending to, and empathizing with another, but is not identical with those ways of relating; I elaborate on these and other distinctions in Section 6.1.3. By claiming that uptake is a virtue, I emphasize its characteristics in terms of the general features of virtue (see Chapter 2). As with other virtues, giving uptake rightly contributes to living well (flourishing, in Aristotle's terms, or aiming for a non-ideal flourishing, in this book's analysis). Giving uptake well is a disposition to attend carefully, actively, and openly to the communication of another. As with other dispositional states, it has to be learned. Aristotle used an analogy with music to explain how virtues are learned. Musical education involves a "mimetic enactment of poetry, song, and dance," whereby the learner comes to feel from within, and learning to be good requires the same internalization of good pleasures and values (Sherman 1989, 182). With respect to giving uptake, we have to learn how and when to listen well, toward whom, and to know why it is important to do this. That is, giving uptake, like other virtues, has a mean and extremes: we can be dialogically responsive either too much and too little, and in both ways not well; we should aim for the intermediate. This chapter describes only the intermediate condition (see Potter 2009, ch. 8, and Potter 2002 for a discussion of the extremes). Additionally, being the sort of person who gives uptake rightly requires that we engage with others richly rather than superficially. By this claim, I mean that we do not hear only words or speech acts, but neither do we freely interpret or impose meanings ourselves. Because it concerns a quality of listening and of grasping another's world, it engages one's social self, with all those meanings, values, advantages, or adversities included, and it requires a shift or decentering of that social self.

As I have said, being the sort of person who gives uptake rightly requires certain sorts of responses, such as attention, recognition, and nonjudgmental receiving of another's communications. This, in turn, requires that we develop epistemic virtue, because uptake is strongly epistemological. One might say that it is a mean between requiring conclusive reasons in order to accept another's communications as true or reasonable, on the one hand, and perfunctorily dismissing, trivializing, discrediting, or ignoring another's communications, on the other hand. Epistemic features of giving uptake include understanding (of the causal history and the social context of the communication); grasping (a deeper level of understanding); openness (to the communicator's credibility, to the possibility that the communicator's perspective is true); and non-defensiveness. In order to give uptake well, the listener needs to be *together with* the communicator in a specific way. This is not a claim that listener and communicator literally need to be in the same room together but, instead, that the listener needs to be oriented toward the communicator with that (epistemic) understanding, grasping, openness, and non-defensiveness. For psychiatrists, who are in a clinical relationship with their patients, giving uptake well emphasizes a relational, or intersubjective, engagement that the listener holds toward the speaker. As such, the relational component makes an ethical demand of the listener. (I will explain in Section 6.1.3 that this is not the same as empathy.) Giving uptake well, therefore, is both epistemological and ethical because it requires *phronesis*—the active engagement of both intellectual and moral character—in order to give uptake well. Giving uptake is a particular sort of stance, an attitude about belief, warrant, and the worth of the communicator in the broader context of the situatedness of both communicator and the listener.

As a virtue, it is intrinsically good. Because we necessarily are interactional and social beings, we unavoidably communicate and respond to one another. It is good and right that we do so well—or as well as we can. Like other virtues, such as justice and friendship, giving uptake is praiseworthy in itself, meaning that it would be choiceworthy even if it did not promote any further good end. But, like other virtues, it is also instrumentally good. I suggest four reasons to think this is the case. First, it is epistemologically necessary for understanding another at a deep level. It does not require that we agree with another's communications, but it does require that we respond in ways that open up and sustain dialogue (within the mean). Doing so allows for the possibility of knowing another person, a core component of good psychiatry (see Introduction). It allows us to grasp, from the other person's perspective, what it is like to be that person, to hold another's values, beliefs, suffering and joy, lived conditions, and world-view. This is important not only to good treatment but also to good diagnosis (including a determination of whether or not a diagnosis is appropriate). Second, giving uptake rightly fosters not only knowledge of, or about, the communicator and his or her values, struggles, insights, and so on, but also self-knowledge. By listening in a certain way, we can come to know ourselves more deeply (if not always easily and comfortably). Consistent with my Aristotelian approach to non-ideal flourishing, giving uptake properly is a quality of being and not just of doing. It is potentially constitutive of rich shifts in self-understanding. Third, giving uptake rightly fosters trust and indicates our trustworthiness. How we respond to another's communications and the degree to which we give uptake to the communicator tells the communicator something about our character. Being trustworthy says to another that I can be counted on to take care of something that person values according to his or her idea of taking care and not mine. Trustworthiness, too, is a virtue, and we can get it wrong about how far to go in staying worthy of another's trust in us. Also, being trustworthy is no guarantee that others will trust us (see Potter 2002). Still, in general, when we give uptake rightly, we will foster trusting relations with others. A fourth reason that the virtue of giving uptake is good to cultivate is that, when we give uptake well, we rectify injustices. As I explained in Section 6.1.1, people who already are disadvantaged or oppressed (such as women of all colors, shapes, and sizes), or the mentally ill, are taken to be less credible—less likely to be reliable witnesses, less reliable narrators, and less likely to be counted as knowers. Thus, they receive uptake less often from people who are positioned in more advantaged or socially privileged positions. (Of course, psychiatrists are not automatically skeptical just because a patient is mentally ill; the degree of uptake depends on the type of communication as it intersects with various symptoms of a particular mental disorder). Nevertheless, as Miranda Fricker argues, some "telling" doesn't get listened to properly (Fricker 2007). This point is pertinent to my discussion of uptake as a virtue because, on Fricker's analysis, to tell is to give testimony, and testimony requires that the listener evaluate the credibility of the speaker as well as the probability that what the communicator tells is true. Without engaging in the qualities needed to give uptake rightly, the weighing of testimony and the types of knowledge that telling conveys are vulnerable to error and distortion. Fricker (2007) analyzes an example from Patricia Highsmith's *The Talented Mr. Ripley* where Marge's fiancé, Dickie, has disappeared. Marge suspects Dickie's friend Tom of being responsible for some evil that has befallen Dickie. Herbert, Dickie's father, dismisses her insights because she is a woman. As Fricker explains,

Herbert constructs Marge as just another hysterical female (Fricker 2007, ch. 4). Fricker calls this a case of testimonial injustice—one form that epistemic injustice takes—where the "hearers fail to exercise any critical awareness regarding the prejudice that is distorting their perception of the speaker" (Fricker 2007, 89).

To be *epistemically unjust* means that the listener could have done otherwise and that his or her failure to attend appropriately to the speaker results in distorted beliefs. It occurs when the listener holds (often socially based) biases and prejudices that influence his or her assessment of the speaker's telling. It is ethically unjust because it is *unfair*: the listener does not accord the speaker the credibility that is warranted, because he or she holds biases and prejudices that influence his or her assessment of the speaker's telling. Marge, then, can be understood to be excluded from what Fricker calls "trustful conversation" (Fricker 2007, 52).

This point applies to many people who behave defiantly. Trustful conversation is one of the ways that the mind steadies itself (Fricker 2007, 52) and, when someone is repeatedly denied testimonial justice—that is, when she or he has a history of not being given uptake—it "gnaws away at a person's intellectual confidence, or never lets it develop in the first place" and damages her or his epistemic function in general (Fricker 2007, 50). This is only one way in which people are damaged when they are not given uptake, but since so much of ordinary life depends on who we believe and what we come to believe in—including people's testimony about economic deprivation and experiences of racism, homophobia, and transphobia—testimonial justice can be said to be a primary virtue to pursue. Giving uptake is a central avenue to fostering such justice. By receiving another's communications with openness, seriousness, and attentiveness, we give uptake to them in ways that can undercut dominant and harmful ways of interacting. One form this takes is in not further entrenching burdened virtues in the communicator. This may seem like an indirect rectification of injustices—and, indeed, it is not enough for long-standing structural injustices to weaken—but it is a constitutive shift in its own right.

6.1.3 Distinguishing uptake from related concepts

A number of terms capture the idea of giving uptake well, such as empathy, validation, attunement, and attention. These concepts are interrelated and, I would argue, are family resemblances. I focus on the first two of these concepts. Concisely defined, empathy is "a complex imaginative process in which an observer simulates another person's situated psychological states while maintaining clear self-other differentiation" (Coplan 2011, 5); Peter

Goldie defines it as a process by which a person centrally imagines the narrative (the thoughts, feelings, and emotions) of another (Goldie 2000); and Jodi Halpern defines it as "an essentially experiential understanding of another person that involves an active, yet not necessarily voluntary, creation of an *interpretive* context" (Halpern 2001, 77; emphasis in original). Uptake is not the same as empathy, but it often includes empathetic feelings and attitudes toward another. Sometimes, but not always, having and expressing empathy toward another facilitates giving that person uptake; at other times, empathy might emerge from giving uptake. Empathy and uptake are distinct virtues, however—empathy is a kind of being-with, while giving uptake is dialogical: it requires a response from the listener that will extend communication and expand meaning and understanding of another, a requirement not constitutive of being empathetic. Uptake can give one a toe-hold to enter more fully into another person's experiential world—that is, more emotionally and more empathetically—and empathy and uptake can be mutually reinforcing, but they call upon different qualities in communicating and understanding another.

Giving uptake is also related to, but not the same as, validating another. We can see a family resemblance with uptake by considering Marcia Linehan's work with patients diagnosed with Borderline Personality Disorder. In defining validation, Linehan says that the therapist "actively accepts the patient," "takes the patient's responses seriously and does not discount or trivialize them"; validation requires that "the therapist search for, recognize, and reflect to the patient" that the patient's communications are understandable and that they make sense in the context of the person's current experience (Linehan 1993, 223–4). Invalidation occurs when the therapist "offers or insists on an interpretation of behavior that is not shared by the patient," ignores important communications or actions of the patient, or "criticizes or punishes the patient's behavior" (Linehan 1993, 76). The purpose of validation is twofold: it honors "the essential wisdom" of the patient, and it develops the capacity for change.

Thus, Linehan's idea of validation sounds a lot like the virtue of giving uptake. Still, uptake and validation are distinct constructs. My concept of uptake is not as strong as validation. By this comment, I mean that giving uptake well does not require that the listener believes the communicator or assumes that he holds "essential wisdom," but only that the listener adopts a stance of openness toward the speaker and a willingness to believe. However, in another sense, giving uptake requires more of the listener than does giving validation. To give uptake rightly, the listener needs to decenter oneself and one's values, meanings, and beliefs while simultaneously attending to what the other communicates. As such, if I understand Linehan correctly, it requires more social, political, and epistemological awareness than does giving validation to another. Additionally, for Linehan, validating another's perspectives, values, beliefs, and feelings should not occur when there is a risk that dysfunctional behavior will be reinforced through validation (Linehan 1993, 226). Throughout this book, however, I have argued that assessing reasonableness and dysfunction is fraught with epistemic and social problems. In sum, validation is related to, but distinct from, uptake.

Giving uptake requires that we do not assume that our ontological and epistemological beliefs about rationality and dysfunction are correct—in fact, it may require that we bracket off those beliefs and assumptions. I have used the term "decentering" as a quality and stance needed in order to give uptake well. Decentering is part of "world"-traveling, a methodology that requires more shifting to another's world and more shifting of one's perspective than other, related concepts do. "World"-traveling, as I described in Section 5.5.2, is needed in order to open themselves to some of the epistemic, social, and ethical challenges raised in this book (see Potter 2003 for more on "world"-traveling).

6.1.4 Application to defiance

Giving uptake well requires that the psychiatrist be attuned to the patient. It involves openness to meaning-making that may be closed off when the psychiatrist employs conventional interpretations of others' communicative acts. It also requires that the psychiatrist is actively engaged in seeking resonance with the patient. This engagement involves the full presence of the psychiatrist with a certain quality of listening. The psychiatrist decenters oneself, while retaining one's self to some degree,

I apply this idea to those on the receiving end of defiance. By giving uptake, the psychiatrist indicates to the patient: you can count on me to take you seriously according to your idea of seriousness and not mine alone; you can expect me to treat your picture of the world seriously and take your defiance seriously. To take defiance seriously is to recognize the call another is making to the listener, a call that often requires the listener to suspend or critically examine norms that he or she is upholding and practices that may not benefit the defiant patient. Taking defiance seriously means that the psychiatrist is willing to consider the possibility that he or she is implicated in reproducing and reinforcing burdened virtues in ways that can be damaging to others. It indicates that the psychiatrist recognizes the worth and dignity of the communicator by being attuned to, and resonating with, the patient's defiance even when the listener does not agree. Typically, it involves granting the communicator a degree of credibility. The psychiatrist does not assume that the defiant one has a mental disorder or that a particular expression of defiance is merely symptomatic. It often involves being open to understanding the broader social context of the patient's lived conditions—such as living with racism, sexism, stigma, poverty, and rigid dichotomies of gender—in order to more fully grasp the meaning of the patient's defiance. Giving uptake to a patient's defiance means that the psychiatrist does not rush to corral passionate expressions of that defiance or to tame it into something more comfortable for the psychiatrist to accept. Lastly, developing a disposition to give uptake rightly means that, when confronted with the defiant behavior of the patient, the psychiatrist reflects not only on the patient's behavior, but also on his or her own assumptions, biases, and world-view. I return to this point in Section 6.4.2.

I now consider how the virtue of giving uptake well plays out in a given clinical encounter. Rachel, as readers may recall from Chapter 3, was outraged with her psychiatrist, Dr. Padgett, because of the way she learned of her diagnosis of Borderline Personality Disorder. She started out with verbal abuse and physical agitations that expressed her fury. Her psychiatrist firmly chastised her abusive approach. He reminded her that she needs to use words instead of body language to communicate with him. Then she did use words: "fuck you." Let's look at how the encounter between Rachel and Dr. Padgett unfolds after she says that.

> Dr. Padgett says "that's not what I'm talking about, and you know it. Cussing me out is just another way of acting out. It doesn't tell me what you feel or why you're feeling it." Rachel feels "the cold slap of having stepped over the line" and is silent. Into this silence, Dr. Padgett says, "Are you listening now? Are you ready to look at this issue now? Is the adult in control?" and he proceeds to explain why he didn't tell her in a way that was easier for Rachel. (Reiland 2004, 123–4)

Now, I do not know all the reasons why Dr. Padgett responds in this way to what I have called Rachel's defiance, and the narrative I am following is Rachel's memoir and thus is her subjective understanding of her treatment with him. So, my analysis here is interpretive based on Rachel's memoir and may not accurately reflect Dr. Padgett's approach or disposition in working with Rachel. Nevertheless, I believe this to be an instructive encounter to examine with respect to the virtue of giving uptake. I believe that Dr. Padgett rightly did not give uptake to Rachel's abusive approach. But something is amiss in this encounter. Rachel comes storming into his office with heightened passions because she feels betrayed by Dr. Padgett and is very frightened about her diagnosis. He immediately works to tame and dampen her passions and continues to do so throughout this encounter, reinforcing the gendered norm that Rachel needs to acquire a virtue that is burdened—the calmed-down, submissive, "good patient" role expected especially of women. Yet even when she behaves as Dr. Padgett demands, she is told that *she* needs to listen. Her defiant behavior is interpreted as regression instead of being taken seriously as a potential offense or harm that her psychiatrist inflicted. Dr. Padgett does not address her anger directly; he does not take responsibility for having hurt her. I suggest that a crucial part of Rachel's continuing anger is that she is not getting uptake. Dr. Padgett is not resonating with Rachel's feelings of betrayal; he is not open to the possibility that she is being defiant of norms and expectations in clinic—and possibility of gender norms for submissiveness in women—and that her defiance may have some merit, albeit not well expressed. He does not listen well himself, instead requiring Rachel to listen to his explanation. It is good that he gives an explanation as to why he handled the delivery of her diagnosis the way he did, but he fails to give uptake to her defiance in a way that does not see it as a mere symptom.

Psychiatrists need to cultivate a number of virtues in order to be good practitioners: they need not only to give uptake properly but also to be empathetic, patient, courageous, and persistent in helping their patients in constructive ways. They need to be trustworthy and just. These and other virtues need to be demonstrated in the therapeutic encounter so that the patient can observe and feel what positive, healthy, and appropriate engagement with another is like. In order to exhibit such virtues, psychiatrists need to practice the virtues even when they are not fully developed in order for them to become habits of intellect and character. Additionally, they need to be effortful in learning to decenter themselves. Finally, as noted in earlier chapters, the psychiatrist–patient relationship is imbued with power differentials that the psychiatrist is expected to handle judiciously. The position of authority that the psychiatrist holds, as in other positions of authority, comes with attendant responsibilities, such as not to abuse that power. Each of these points is relevant to the virtue of giving uptake, as many of these and other virtues are called upon when giving uptake to patients. The virtues work together, as Aristotle says, and are mutually reinforcing, enhancing one another as they are cultivated and expressed.

I have argued that one of the virtues is that of giving uptake, and that being the sort of person who does this well is praiseworthy. I also have argued that giving uptake is a central virtue for psychiatrists to cultivate and have described what it would look like in relation to defiance. However, giving uptake well is difficult to do well. In Section 6.2, I discuss some reasons why it can be difficult that go beyond individual foibles and failings.

6.2 **Knowing, ignoring, and resisting knowledge**

Throughout this book, I have emphasized the social realities of domination and subordination, and of structural advantage and disadvantage, as they relate to how defiant behavior can be interpreted and responded to. In this section, I focus on the field of epistemology (what knowledge is and what is required to be a knower) in order to explain more fully why giving uptake is difficult and what might be involved in learning to give uptake well to defiant people. I introduce a particular way of understanding knowledge, knowing, and knowers, and why we may have what I'll call "willful ignorance" about some things and about some people, including ourselves. I first describe this way of thinking about the process of knowing, called social epistemology, and then I explain a particular set of concerns that some social epistemologists identify. After this discussion, I apply these theories to psychiatry. In Section 6.3, I analyze another example in light of the discussion in Section 6.2.

6.2.1 **Social epistemology**

Epistemology in Western philosophy standardly has been understood as an individualist enterprise—that is, each of us comes to know that others' claims about knowledge and knowing are true by adopting an objective, detached, and disinterested stance. Social epistemology developed as a theory that more accurately describes how people come to know things; it locates the individual knowledge-seeker within social groups and positionalities within hierarchies. As Charles Mills says, the development of social epistemology is a welcome change (Mills 2007). Many social epistemologists claim that bodies of knowledge always are created by groups of knowers who jointly decide what will count as knowledge and who the knowers are within a given field of knowledge (such as the field of jazz music or of fair treatment in racial profiling). Social epistemologists argue that the production of knowledge is not just a fact-based examination of knowledge claims that individuals (usually experts in a given field) either consider justified or wrong-headed, but a social enterprise that involves people in deciding what will count as evidence and what the standards for assessment should be. Lynn Hankinson Nelson makes a stronger claim about knowers and knowledge in her theorizing of social epistemology and epistemic communities. She argues that communities, not individuals, are the primary "generators, repositories, holders, and acquirers of knowledge" (Nelson 1993).

> In suggesting that it is communities that construct and acquire knowledge, I do not mean (or "merely" mean) that what comes to be recognized or "certified" as knowledge is the result of collaborations between, consensus achieved by, political

struggles engaged in, negotiations undertaken among, or other activities engaged in by individuals who, *as individuals, know* in some logically or empirically "prior" sense. Work in sociology of knowledge, feminist epistemology and philosophy of science, and social studies of science indicates that it is in and through a variety of such activities that knowledge is generated. The change I am proposing involves what we should construe as the *agents* of these activities. My arguments suggest that the collaborators, the consensus achievers, and, in more general terms, the agents who generate knowledge are communities and subcommunities, not individuals. (Nelson 1993; emphasis in original)

Nelson's claim that the agents of knowing activities are communities and not individuals is important because, in thinking about how psychiatrists learn to know, what they assume to be true about behavior and dysfunction, and how they might challenge the current psychiatric practices, it is the *episteme* of psychiatry that needs to be targeted. This is not to say that psychiatrists do not treat individuals, but, instead, that patients need to be seen as knowers of local and situated knowledge (see Chapters 4 and 5) and that, as an institutionalized practice, they will be better positioned to give uptake rightly to defiant patients if they critically engage with—or even reconceptualize—their own knowing practices. In order to motivate this claim, I first will lay the groundwork by discussing *epistemes* more generally. The term *episteme* comes from the Greek and is translated as "knowledge" but has been broadened by twentieth-century philosophers to apply to the knowledge base that shapes a given practice within a particular period of time. In describing the force of *epistemes* to shape character formation, I turn to a newer development in social epistemology—one that focuses on what, at first, might seem to be an oxymoron: epistemologies of ignorance.

6.2.2 **Epistemologies of ignorance**

Epistemologies of ignorance are one of the stubborn and entrenched ways that members of dominant, powerful, or privileged groups maintain power. They are practices of willful ignorance. As such, they not only involve the dissemination of misinformation, but also a habit of knowing only in a certain way, and about particular things and not others, and in an interested and invested manner. (In other words, this is not the stuff of knowledge as discovered by detached, disinterested, and objective knowers, as traditional epistemology has proclaimed.) Epistemologies of ignorance have an ordinariness to them that belies the technical term I have used here. In reality, they are the everyday "gaps" in knowledge that can be actively produced and sustained for the purposes of maintaining social patterns of domination and exploitation (Alcoff 2007). For example, most people in wealthier countries take for granted that the garbage will be picked up on time, but those who are advantaged may ignore the reality of the work entailed in being a person who picks up others' trash. The idea behind willful ignorance is that many of the things that privileged people "don't know" take effort; it isn't accidental that some people remain ignorant about the realities of historical and persistent systematic oppressions. I do not mean that willful ignorance necessarily is conscious and deliberate. It is important both to be aware of the way domination and advantages are reproduced intentionally and to attend to the ways that even good intentions can reproduce systemically adverse conditions unintentionally: that is, even unintentional harms may be culpably produced and reproduced.

Theories of not-knowing and not-needing-to-know focus on whether or not ignorance could be avoided and what the ignorant person or group of persons does to allow or maintain that ignorance. This way of thinking about responsible ignorance is consistent with Aristotle's distinction between blameworthy and accidental ignorance. Drawing on an Aristotelian theory of moral responsibility, I argue that it is not enough to avoid culpability for wrong actions for someone to claim that he or she is ignorant of the effects of our beliefs, attitudes, policies, norms, and actions; the questions one needs to consider are whether one could have known, and to actively engage in critical and honest examination about how one might be contributing to not-knowing—and how one's own not-knowing might be complicit in maintaining structures of oppression and systematic harms.

Linda Alcoff analyzes the role that dominant epistemic norms play in maintaining the belief that society is basically just, despite evidence to the contrary. She argues for the need within dominant groups to develop cognitive norms that enable people to dismiss the countervailing evidence and maintain the fiction of living in a basically just world (Alcoff 2007, 48). These cognitive norms are supported and maintained by the phenomenon called confirmation bias, which is defined as "the inappropriate bolstering of hypotheses or beliefs whose truth is in question" (Nickerson 1998, 175). Confirmation bias is found in psychiatry (Mendel et al. 2011), the criminal justice system (Ditrich 2015), and the educational system (Podell and Soodak 1993), not to mention everyday life. As Raymond Nickerson describes it, confirmation bias is selective one-sided case-building to bolster one's position, hypothesis, or theory, and it is widely recognized as one of the most common errors of inferential reasoning (Nickerson 1998). However, calling it an error may be too generous when it comes to practices of willful ignorance: confirmation bias allows one to ignore evidence that the world we live in is unjust and that injustice is not natural, inevitable, or accidental. While cognitive bias is a problem for most (if not all) people, it takes an especially egregious form when coupled with dominant cognitive norms of willful ignorance. An example of this is the practice of color-blindness, which perpetuates racial injustice (Mills 2010). Mills argues that this practice denies the differential positioning of Blacks and whites and denies that a system exists which structures such advantages and disadvantages (Mills 2010, 362). Color-blindness, Mills argues, is:

> key to this mystification and obfuscation of social reality, and needs to be identified and criticized as such. For what it really expresses is a willed blindness to, a refusal to see, the enduring structures of white privilege, in terms of income, wealth, educational opportunity, residential advantage, likelihood of imprisonment, differential life-expectancy, and numerous other factors. (Mills 2010, 362)

The ideology of color-blindness reinforces and reproduces social injustices and adverse conditions. By relying on epistemic ignorance, color-blindness forecloses alternative interpretations, analyses, and critique of existing structures of racial discrimination and racialized social injustices. To specify one effect: it forecloses the possibility of giving uptake well to people's communications about racial injustice.

The connection between giving uptake well and theories about willful ignorance is that epistemologies of ignorance are likely to be part of the training and habituating of privileged and advantaged people. As earlier chapters have suggested, we learn what it means to be successful (satisfied, accepted, and so on) through learning habits and norms about who we are and what we do. This affects our ability, and even our interest and willingness, to learn to give uptake well. In thinking about training and habituation in terms of *epistemes*, I see "being" and "doing" not merely as actions performed by individuals but as expressions of struggles to situate groups favorably and to situate other groups as disadvantaged. As part of being habituated into adulthood, epistemologies of ignorance, like maturation in general, are an ongoing task of learning to become the sort of person one is in relation to one's status, social positionings, and location in hierarchies of power/knowledge. This education, like the Aristotelian idea of learning to be virtuous and to take pleasure in what is good and fine, is both epistemic and ethical: we come to "know" what is good as well as what is true. Yet the sort of education into epistemic ignorance is not one of virtues but of vices. As we saw with respect to color-blindness, this training allows white people to believe in a just, equitable, and merit-based world even while evidence is abundantly available that counters such beliefs. When we come to see that practices of not-knowing and willful ignorance are structural and that they benefit members of dominant groups, we are better able to see that those benefitting from structural epistemic ignorance may have internalized patterns of belief-forming practices that sustain harmful effects. Through patterns of social reward, moral development, and training of civil behavior, members of dominant groups may be forming knowledge that is "actively pursuing or supporting a distorted or an otherwise inaccurate account" (Alcoff 2007, 48).

Although harmful epistemologies may be quite generalized to social structures, there is no one overarching *episteme*. Although she frames her discussion in terms of cultures instead of *epistemes*, Michele Moody-Adams also talks about habituation as the process of learning the cultural norms about emotions, thought, and actions that give particular shape to a group's practices (Moody-Adams 1994, 295). She, too, rejects the idea that, because we are socialized into particular norms and practices, we cannot be held accountable for wrong or harmful practices. That is an epistemic claim that implies that ignorance is a moral excuse. But the fact that a culture accepts an internal perspective on its rules and norms does not mean that it, or the people within it, cannot critically reflect and question, or even reject, those norms and rules. So, when a culture accepts its own norms, it is more a matter of "choosing not to know what one can and should know ... refusing to consider whether some practice in which one participates might be wrong" (Moody-Adams 1994, 296). Ignorance can be dangerously self-deceptive and self-interested.

Epistemologies of ignorance, therefore, impede our ability to give uptake well. This difficulty applies to all or most people, but it does not apply equally. That is, people who have a stake in preserving the status quo, with its material, legal, educational, and social advantages, especially may find it difficult both to develop dispositions to listen well and openly to those in disadvantaged positions and to make shifts that would allow for better uptake to be given. The point is that giving uptake well has consequences—sometimes material, social, and legal ones that advantaged people unconsciously or deliberately may be reluctant to accept. I will explain how this applies to psychiatrists, who have the best interests of their patients at heart, in Section 6.3. Then, in Section 6.4, I illustrate how these theories apply to giving uptake to a defiant patient.

6.2.3 Epistemologies of resistance

Another way to ascertain why giving uptake is difficult to do well is by turning to what José Medina, who analyzes both the force of epistemic intransigence and the possibility for change, calls epistemologies of resistance. In brief, Medina argues that differentially situated people form resistances that shape the experiences one has, the kinds of concepts one forms, and the beliefs one holds about what is true about the world (Mills, as quoted in Medina 2013, 48). These resistances form the trajectory of belief-formation and the external forces that steer the course of epistemic character development in differentially situated people (Medina 2013, 48).

Epistemic resistances, in their various forms of not-knowing, are dispositional tendencies that people in situations of privilege develop as they attempt to reduce epistemic friction and hold on to the confidence of their positions as knowers. Because these resistances become part of our character, they are also metaphysical. By this I mean that they become a deep part of our being in the sense that they are a way of relating to others—both the in-groups and the out-groups (see Cudd 2006). As such, epistemic resistances become stubborn, entrenched, and difficult to change as they run deep within our embodied sense of ourselves and others, and express our most fundamental orientation and quality of relationality toward others. I will focus on resistances that members of advantaged groups develop as part of their character. Medina is careful to emphasize that there is no simple equation between privilege and epistemic vice on the one hand, and oppression and epistemic virtue on the other hand. As he says, we cannot determine a person's epistemic character just by identifying the social position of that person. The point is that systems of oppression and domination create *patterns* that are found in these different social groupings.

Consistent with my framework for virtue theory, Medina argues that epistemic flaws are grounded in and exhibit our character (Medina 2013, 29). Vices and virtues are not temporary or one-off flaws or strengths but are partly constitutive of who we are and how we perceive, respond to, and help shape the world and the various people within it. Thus, they are not only individual flaws or strengths, but also systemic and structural ones: epistemology is a social endeavor that involves others in deciding what counts as knowledge and knowers, and so on. Cognitive and social development work together to cultivate our epistemic schemas for navigating the world—schemas that simultaneously create our characters. These schemas or blueprints shape our bodies of knowledge: who we count as knowers, what we count as evidence, who we count as credible, and who determines the structure of various practices. These schemas may not be conscious but they still can impede our giving uptake properly. Although we typically are not aware of our everyday attitudes, beliefs, and assumptions, and usually are not critically evaluating our own epistemic frameworks, we are responsible for them because we *can* be critically aware, we *can* evaluate and change our own epistemic character, and we *can* learn to understand who we are and who others are in a more epistemically and socially accurate way. We *can* engage in strong objectivity, both in science and in ethics. And because epistemic vices are integrally tied to social injustice, we not only *can*, but *should* make the necessary cognitive corrections in order to cultivate more virtuous characters. Thus, Medina argues that one form epistemic character flaws take is a resistance to self-correction and openness to correction from others (Medina 2013, 31). This is a vice when it becomes a habit, part of our disposition, because "letting one's perspective go unchecked results in an unavoidable, mundane accumulation of oversights, errors, biased stereotypes, and distortions. In this way, racist and sexist biases become undetectable and incorrigible blind spots" (Medina 2013, 32):

> Being sensitive to the presence and influence of cognitive forces is crucial to the achievement of epistemic virtues. . .the willingness to put one's cognitive perspective in relation to that of others—calibrating the different cognitive forces, impulses, and compulsions one is exposed to—is the path to the epistemic virtues. (Medina 2013, 51)

Although Medina is talking about epistemic virtues in the oppressed in this passage, he also applies the normative claim to the privileged. Regardless of where we are situated in relation to structures of domination and subordination, we need to develop a character with epistemic virtues in order to serve social justice and fight against injustice. But the road to epistemic virtue is, in many ways, more challenging and more difficult for the privileged. In particular, it presents a challenge to psychiatrists and other mental health professionals.

Medina's work suggests that the project of change is substantial and difficult:

> Active ignorance has deep psychological and sociopolitical roots: it is supported by psychological structures and social arrangements that prevent subjects from correcting misconceptions and acquiring knowledge because they would have to change so much of themselves and their communities before they can start seeing things differently. (Medina 2013, 58)

These resistances are active, even though they may not be deliberate. For example, as Medina says, "there is *not needing to know* and *needing not to know*" (Medina 2013, 34; emphasis in original). Needing not to know, in his view, is a defense mechanism, a kind of epistemic hiding that functions to preserve privilege. It is a culpable form of ignorance and, if it becomes part of one's character, it is a vice. As with other vices, it becomes embedded in our personal, social, and economic histories, and is life-directing, action-guiding, and meaning-making. Epistemic resistances, therefore, entail certain ontological-assumptive values. As John Sadler explains, ontological values "concern commitments to particular notions of human nature; the structure and organization of the self; intersubjectivity; notions about space, time, and causality; and other dimensions of human experience and being" (Sadler 2005, 38; see also Sadler 2005, section 5.3). Epistemic resistances entail presuppositions about how the world is and ought to be—presuppositions that are then subject to confirmation bias and, often, willful ignorance.

For example, inattention to intersectionalities, as I discussed in Chapter 4, would be said to involve actively embracing one's own positionality without attending either to self-knowledge or to knowledge of other persons with their own historically and socially situated backgrounds, experiences, values, and beliefs. The epistemic character flaw here is that it assumes that there is nothing to see and that another's historical and social situatedness is not significant (Medina 2013, 38). One's character is that of an actively ignorant subject; actively ignorant subjects are

> those who can be blamed not just for lacking particular pieces of knowledge, but also for having epistemic habits and attitudes that contribute to create and maintain bodies of ignorance. These subjects are at fault for their complicity (often unconscious and involuntary) with epistemic injustices that support and contribute to situations of oppression. (Medina 2013, 39)

That passage, and the argument about epistemic ignorance and resistance overall, may tend to put readers on the defensive. Yet, it is not my intention to cast readers as blameworthy in these ways, but to motivate them to think critically about what they have internalized about knowing and knowers, and about how such internalized and dispositional schemas affect their ability to give uptake rightly. The point of all this theorizing is to apply some of these insights to psychiatric practices.

6.3 **Epistemology and psychiatry**

Psychiatrists, too, are socialized into epistemic communities. This epistemic socialization involves an "implicit consensus about cognitive norms, it concerns what counts as a correct interpretation of the world, and what actions are right and legal in it" (Bailey 2007, 79). As I argue elsewhere,

> the *episteme* in psychiatry includes ontological commitments about what exists in the world: mental disorders exist; they exist as biological entities; causal explanations of mental disorders are located in brain sciences; causal explanations that refer back to spirits, ancestors, or folk magic do not. It follows from these ontological commitments that pathologies in cognition, affect, and behavior exist: people's reasoning may be distorted not just in ordinary ways but in psychotic ways; their affect may be dysregulated; their behavior may be dysfunctional. (Potter 2015)

One way that the psychiatric *episteme* organizes its epistemology and grounds ontological commitments is through the DSM. A central task of psychiatry is to delineate the lines between normal and abnormal. Psychiatrists, along with other parts of the health care team, are the primary knowers; they are the experts. As such, they interpret people's presentation, their body language, their stories, and their behavior according to a given world-view. They draw upon the whole of the psychiatric *episteme*, including beliefs, medical education, and personal habituation, in order to delineate and distinguish between a sick person and a well one. In this way, psychiatrists hold the authority to decide that some people are "patients" and that some may be a danger to themselves or others. This authoritative responsibility within the *episteme* prepares them to have their interpretive lens be determined at least in part, and often significantly, by current best practices as defined primarily by Evidence-Based Medicine; although they may take in the social dimensions of a patient's life as it bears on diagnosis and treatment, most psychiatrists are trained to bracket off the broader cultural and historical context in which persons are situated and immersed. Speaking generally, then, I argue that the *episteme* of psychiatry shapes diagnostic and treatment practices by enculturating practitioners into a specific ontological, evidentiary, and expertise-based way of knowing what to pay attention to and how to interpret things. Like other institutions of privilege and power, psychiatry inculcates in its practice such resistance to certain bodies of knowledge that can affect psychiatrists' character and, hence, their diagnoses.

Psychiatrists do not embody and sustain the *episteme* of psychiatry all by themselves. Patients are part of this *episteme* (for example, by enacting the good patient role or being compliant even when they believe they should be defiant). However, my aim in this chapter is to motivate psychiatrists to take seriously the way that willful ignorance and resistance to knowledges function in their lives and the lives of those people whom they encounter in their practices. At the same time, I hope that service users will find resonance with my argument that defiance sometimes is a virtue. The point is that problematic epistemologies can implicate psychiatrists and the institution of psychiatry in ways that harm others—especially disadvantaged others and those living in adverse conditions. While a central aspect and value within psychiatry is a conception of itself as a helping profession, with emphasis on the ideal of being helpers and healers, I argue that the *episteme* of psychiatry habituates and trains many, if not most, psychiatrists epistemically, ethically, and socio-politically such that they are the authoritative body about what counts as mental health and how to respond to problems in mental health. Often unwittingly, but nevertheless with willful ignorance, this *episteme* runs the risk of being part of the reproduction of harms to some of those most affected by the historical and current context of interlocking oppression, domination, and systematic injustices. Specific to this book's central thesis on defiance, the psychiatric *episteme* may encourage ignorance of the possibility of righteous and reasonable defiance against hegemonic power.

Such dispositional tendencies are a vulnerability for psychiatrists and other mental health professionals because their training, as well as the emphasis on Evidence-Based Medicine and the role of the DSM, often work together to create clinicians with an epistemology of resistance to the historical and socially situated persons with whom they come into contact. That is, they are expected—indeed, may even be required—to narrowly focus on the person as a generic individual as they decide whether to diagnose or not. It is true that the DSM-5 allows for more attention to the social self than previous versions but, as I say, the DSM works together with other epistemic practices that constrict many clinicians' access to knowing well. Thus, clinicians shape themselves into, and are shaped into, a privileged way of knowing that elides many crucial factors that influence the experiences and needs of the person in front of them.

As I say, the DSM does not sustain willful ignorance in isolation. Sadler argues that the DSM is sustained because it plays a role within a broader set of economic and other social and institutional forces—what he calls the "Mental Health Medical Industrial Complex" (MHMIC) (Sadler 2013). "The DSM has prevailed because it has, on balance, served its function in the MHMIC, whose monolithic influences on funding, public policy, and the social discourse on mental illness reinforces the DSM's stability and success" (Sadler 2013, 24). Figure 6.2 schematizes the relations between these forces.

My point is that the broader *episteme* of psychiatry creates scaffolds that support and sustain the DSM and its ways of conceptualizing patients, their behaviors, and their illnesses. Education into and training for becoming a psychiatrist occurs within this context—a context in which psychiatrists are vulnerable to the reinforcement of socially structured willful ignorance, not-knowing, and resistances to knowing even while they also learn about the virtues that are needed to be a good psychiatrist (such as empathy, patience, and so on).

Epistemic ignorance and resistances of the kind I have been discussing affect the perception and interpretation of behavior that may end up being mistaken. Epistemic ignorance and resistances affect one's capacity to hear and to be heard correctly. But being seen and heard correctly are of central importance to good practices in psychiatry and other mental health practices. The social position of privileged people, including that of psychiatrists, affords them the ability not to know certain things and the assumption that they do not need to know certain things—gaps in knowing that affect diagnosis and treatment of patients.

It can be difficult to see how psychiatrists can make changes. Nevertheless, *epistemes* are not totalizing, and epistemologies of ignorance and resistances

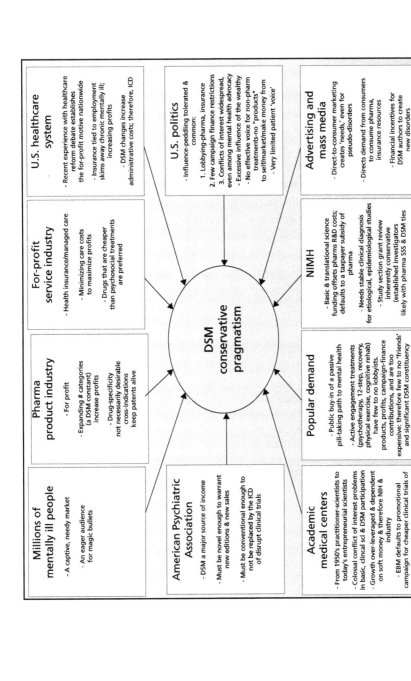

Millions of mentally ill people
- A captive, needy market
- An eager audience for magic bullets

Pharma product industry
- For profit
- Expanding # categories (a DSM constant) increase profits
- Drug-specificity not necessarily desirable cross-indications keep patents alive

For-profit service industry
- Health insurance/managed care
- Minimizing care costs to maximize profits
- Drugs that are cheaper than psychosocial treatments are preferred

U.S. healthcare system
- Recent experience with healthcare reform debate establishes the for-profit motive nationwide
- Insurance tied to employment skims away chronic mentally ill; increasing profits
- DSM changes increase administrative costs; therefore, ICD

American Psychiatric Association
- DSM a major source of income
- Must be novel enough to warrant new editions & new sales
- Must be conventional enough to not be replaced by the ICD of disrupt clinical trials

DSM conservative pragmatism

U.S. politics
- Influence-peddling tolerated & common:
  1. Lobbying-pharma, insurance
  2. Few campaign finance restrictions
  3. Conflicts of interest widespread, even among mental health advocacy
- Excessive influence of the wealthy
- No effective voice for non-pharm treatments–no "products" to self/market/make money from
- Very limited patient 'voice'

Academic medical centers
- From 1950's practitioner-scientists to today's entrepreneurial scientists
- Colossal conflict of interest problems in basic, clinical sci & DSM participation
- Growth over-leveraged & dependent on soft money & therefore NIH & industry
- EBM defaults to promotional campaign for cheaper clinical trials of drug Rx

Popular demand
- Public buy-in of a passive pill-taking path to mental health
- Active engagement treatments (psychotherapy, 12-step, recovery, physical exercise, cognitive rehab) have few to no lobbyists.
- Products, profits, campaign-finance contributions, and are too expensive: therefore few to no "friends' and significant DSM constituency

NIMH
- Basic & translational science funding offsets pharms R&D costs; defaults to a taxpayer subsidy of pharma
- Needs stable clinical diagnosis for etiological, epidemiological studies
- Study section grant review inherently conservative (established investigators likely with pharma SSS & DSM ties

Advertising and mass media
- Direct-to-consumer marketing creates 'needs,' even for pseudo-disorders
- Directs demand from consumers to consume pharma, insurance resources
- Financial incentives for DSM authors to create new disorders

Fig. 6.2 Elements of the MHMIC.

do not always "take." If this were not the case, there would be little point to this theorizing or an analysis of the psychiatric *episteme*. Section 6.4 presents a case study and discussion that illustrates some ways to engage the material presented in this chapter.

6.4 **Case study**

Many members of representative institutions are well-intended and good-hearted; yet, even so, some encounters are, or are experienced by patients, as oppressive. Additionally, some people whose behavior is defiant, or taken to be defiant, are not given uptake well. I have suggested that a core reason why these things happen is that epistemic ignorance and resistance occur, and that the problems attendant with ignorance and resistance need to be addressed. Indeed, without giving uptake rightly, patients may respond in these very psychiatric encounters in a defiant way, so that the psychiatric *episteme* and the training of psychiatrists' dispositions may sometimes even *produce* defiance. These may be difficult claims to accept. Taking these challenges seriously may involve the gentle prodding of readers—and *by* readers—into examining the not-so-benign subtexts of encounters with defiant patients.

6.4.1 **Vignette**

The case I present for discussion is a composite of a patient in the context of an emergency room.

> Jewell, a coffee-colored woman in her early twenties, is brought in to meet with the psychiatric team because she has been kicked out of the half-way house she has been living in. She reports that she has left there voluntarily because she hates it, it is "crazy unreasonable" and that "no one should have to follow that many rules." She appears distressed and agitated. When members of the psychiatric team ask her to explain what is wrong with the place she came from, she becomes angry, saying "I. Already. Told. You." Psychiatrists and others explain that they want her to consider going back there and that she will need to abide by those rules, but that they are "good rules." She stands up and starts pacing back and forth, "There's too many rules! I can't live that way!" When the psychiatric team explains that they believe it is the right place for her and that it will be better for her to learn to follow rules, she shouts, "You people don't understand!" Upon being asked to take a seat so this can be discussed calmly and reasonably, she leaves the room, slamming the door. (Potter 2015)

6.4.2 **Discussion**

As I see it, Jewell defies the rules and norms of the half-way house, and then she defies norms for patient behavior (compliant behavior) in the emergency room. Members of the team discuss what would be the best thing to do for this patient. Yet all of them see her as displaying tendencies of personality disorder and other symptoms of mental disorder—symptoms that, if accurately identified, would explain why Jewell's ability to follow rules is impeded. The discussion centered on tendencies toward antisocial behavior. She was diagnosed tentatively with "personality disorder, not otherwise specified."

What was not discussed was the fact that Jewell was the only Black person in the room. Everyone on the health care team was white.

I have argued in this book that norms for compliant behavior for patients in psychiatry include that the patient does not exhibit defiant or threatening behavior. Behavior such as Jewell's—of not staying seated, of shouting and interrupting the psychiatric team—can be interpreted as defiant and threatening. Yet I call attention to two intersecting issues at play in interpreting and diagnosing Jewell's behavior. The first issue is that psychiatry is ontologically committed to mental disorders as occurring in individuals and is increasingly biologically oriented. Jewell and other patients are likely to be viewed primarily as individuals whose social identity (e.g., intersectional race, class, and gender) typically are not taken into account when trying to understand their behavior. My concern is that the broader historical context of our complex and situated lives may be overlooked, ignored, or erased. I do not mean to suggest that Jewell could not be struggling with mental distress; so, the second issue I call attention to is that, as long as a patient's background social group identity, including intersectionalities, are bracketed off, psychiatrists face the challenging task of identifying which behaviors require psychiatric diagnosis and intervention and which are appropriately defiant. I suggest that the fact that intersectionality is the context of Jewell's life and her presentation in the emergency room is crucial to grasp in order to understand Jewell and to give uptake rightly to her defiance. Therefore, one of the issues that arises when considering the case of Jewell in the earlier vignette is that a racialized patient may be diagnosed with defiant, antisocial behavior without taking into account two things: first, how racialization affects the development of the person she is now; and second, how an epistemology of ignorance may prevent the psychiatrist from properly situating the person's behavior in the context of that racialized background, development, and experience.

Despite the enormous risks involved in being defiant—as manifested in the case of Jewell and, more generally, as discussed in Chapter 4—it sometimes is the appropriate response when facing authoritative bodies such as the schools and psychiatry. Jewell, for instance, may be responding defiantly to norms and expectations from the health care team that she sit quietly, civilly, and circumspectly, and that she ultimately agree to return to the half-way house. Jewell may perceive rightly that the roomful of white folks trained in the psychiatric *episteme* are imposing standards for behavior that fail to account for her experiences as an oppressed racialized woman who is constantly expected to conform to whitely dominant norms for behavior. Jewell may be defiant because she has reached a breaking point with demands that she subordinate herself; she may need to preserve her self-worth *on her terms*. Again, this is not to dismiss the possibility that she may also be dealing with mental distress that needs intervention. My aim is for readers to consider why Jewell might be acting defiantly from her own point of view and within her frame of reference as a racialized woman and to not close off the possibility that her defiance may not be symptomatic and diagnostic. If my argument is on the right track, the central question of this chapter is how psychiatrists should respond when faced with (apparently) defiant patients. The psychiatric *episteme* can powerfully impede accurate understanding of an oppressed person where an historical legacy interacts with current systemic oppressions. But it is from *within that context* that defiant behavior can be more accurately understood.

If we are to listen properly, in a way that genuinely gives uptake to the communicator, it is not enough for the psychiatrist to encounter the patient as "an individual with a mental disorder"—even if this seems to be done with good will and respect—nor is it enough to assume that someone who is defying dominant norms is "acting out"—even if this seems to be done with good will and concern.

I suggest seven things:

1. situate the person within her or his social context;
2. situate the person within her or his historical context, which context will often include oppression, colonization, and transgenerational trauma;
3. know enough about epistemologically harmful strategies to critically engage with them on a structural level as well as within the patient/psychiatrist encounter;
4. educate oneself about what practices of willful ignorance and resistances to responsible knowing are and how they work to maintain hegemonic relations;
5. decenter the self and, in doing so, "world"-travel to the patient's world;
6. critically examine one's own taken-for-granted beliefs and knowledge gaps that benefit dominant power structures, and strategize how to combat them; and
7. prioritize pedagogical efforts to make these dispositional changes possible.[5]

The DSM-5 acknowledges that the first point is relevant to diagnosis and treatment (DSM-5 2013, 724). The introduction to the section in the DSM-5 called "Other Conditions That May Be a Focus of Clinical Attention" makes clear that such conditions as "acculturation difficulty" and "target of (perceived) adverse discrimination or persecution" should not be considered mental disorders, but instead regarded as additional information in the practice of diagnosing, treating, medicating, and ordering tests. Still, the space devoted to each of these social background factors is minimal. Additionally, as I have noted, the nosological structure of psychiatry is grounded firmly in a biologically based and individualist construct of psychopathology. Therefore, the acknowledgment that individuals always live within a social context does little to shift those ontological commitments. It is a pedagogical uncertainty whether or not residents are taught the value, significance, and ontological assumptions behind social factors.

Thus, if psychiatrists are to situate patients in their social context, it is likely that they will need to be personally motivated to do so beyond what the DSM states. Numbers two through six (above) are even more likely to require the initiative of the morally and politically committed to do on their own. This book has emphasized the importance of psychiatric engagement with the complex issue of defiance, and in this chapter I have applied my theory of the virtue of giving uptake as one way for psychiatrists to engage at a richer and more productive level with defiant people. Here, I stress the value of engaging with other like-minded psychiatrists, consistent with the ideas of social epistemology I presented. Given that knowledge-production is not an individual enterprise, and that, from an ecological perspective, knowers are not only those with sociopolitical status or training as experts but are located in ordinary people and at grass-roots levels, knowing well and giving uptake rightly require a pragmatic reconceptualization of who counts as knowers and how knowledge is produced. This is a normative claim in that it holds that epistemically responsible knowledge-production and the development of giving uptake rightly in psychiatry requires a broad engagement with others—not only other psychiatrists, but patients as well. This kind of engagement may require that psychiatrists place themselves in uncomfortable situations where their values, ontological commitments, and world-views may be challenged and they are viewed with distrust (cf. Lugones and Spelman 1983). Doing this can be both enlightening and upsetting, and is likely to call upon the virtues of courage and humility as well as that of giving uptake—in this case, the active engagement of unlearning, giving uptake to those who would challenge them. Importantly, such activity and engagement may be psychiatrists' own form of defiance.

Number seven states that shifts in the *episteme* and practices of psychiatry require pedagogical interventions in residency. For this, I would suggest a course that directly teaches giving uptake as I have analyzed it. Such a course would include discussions of "world"-traveling and would examine some of the assumptions that undergird the *episteme* of psychiatry. This opens up a space for residents to engage in critical reflection of themselves, their beliefs, their values, and their practices. It positions residents to respond well when they encounter problems in behavior—in this book, defiance. However, in order to be effective, this training needs to be woven into other settings and not contained within one course. This, in turn, would call for psychiatric settings to be open to psychiatrists' explorations of shifting their place in the *episteme* and practicing psychiatry differently. Pedagogical changes such as I suggest present an ideal at which to aim. It would not be easy.

The vignette in Section 6.5 illustrates what giving uptake looks like when the psychiatrist begins to critique the psychiatric *episteme* and counter-strategies of epistemology.

6.5 How the analysis of this book might work

Given the analysis of this chapter, it will be clear that being open to understanding and interpreting defiant behavior as a potential virtue can present a significant challenge to psychiatrists. This book argues for a complex and deep understanding of defiance that includes an understanding of how burdened virtues are constituted and how people experience psychiatric disabilities, intersectionalities, authoritative bodies, others' constructions of them as credible or not credible, norms of civility, and norms of practical reasoning. Here, I present a constructed case through which I hope to illustrate some of the key struggles and successes offered by the analysis in this book. I assume a level of epistemic engagement by the psychiatrist, Dr. B, which engagement positions her to give uptake well enough when presented with the patient's defiant behavior. I do not pretend to address all the nuances of a psychiatric encounter here but only to demonstrate what it would look like for a psychiatrist to grapple with the ideas in this book.

> Dolores is a 31-year-old American-born Latina woman. She has been referred to a psychiatrist by her primary care physician, Dr. H, who is concerned that Dolores may be psychotic. Dr. H reports that the patient seems to be paranoid and confused and that she makes threatening remarks about one of her neighbors. Dr. H thinks that Dolores may be dangerous and wants her to be evaluated for treatment options. Dolores adamantly does not want to see a psychiatrist, so Dr. H takes out a court-ordered psychiatric evaluation. Dolores is brought in by local police to see Dr. B.

> Dr. B is a white female psychiatrist who has been involved with a small consciousness-raising group of fellow psychiatrists who want to challenge themselves and each other and to self-reflect about assumptions, beliefs, and attitudes that impede them from using their expertise and medical authority in genuinely helpful ways for patients. When Dolores is brought in to see Dr. B, Dolores remains standing by the

door and against the wall. She uses a loud and frenetic voice, saying there is nothing wrong with her and that her [white] neighbors have "cooked this up" so that she will be silenced. Flailing her arms about, she exclaims that she will not be silenced. She appears angry and frightened.

Dr. B invites Dolores to sit down but does not pressure her to do so. When Dolores remains standing by the door, Dr. B asks her if she would be comfortable with Dr. B standing also. Dolores shrugs, which Dr. B takes to be an indication that it would be acceptable and she stands, leaving some space between them. Dr. B tells Dolores that she is open to believing that Dolores may be suspicious of her neighbors for good reasons, that it is possible that Dolores has experienced racism at their hands. Dr. B invites Dolores to explain how neighbor relations have unfolded from her perspective. Dolores refuses to cooperate, shouting at Dr. B that she does not want to be there. She pulls out a cigarette. Dr. B says that there is no smoking in the building; Dolores lights up anyway. When Dr. B firmly states that Dolores must put out her cigarette immediately, Dolores blows smoke at her, drops her cigarette on the floor, and steps on it to put it out. Dr. B believes that Dolores is being defiant by refusing to sit down and by lighting a cigarette after being told not to. She speculates that Dolores might be expressing defiance to signify her refusal to see Dr. B, a white doctor, as authoritative or as knowledgeable about race relations, let alone capable of understand how racism affects Dolores. Dr. B also realizes that these behaviors may indicate disordered personality tendencies. However, she gives significance to the interpretation that Dolores' defiance may be a proper response to a situation Dolores sees as unequal and threatening to her well-being. Dr. B reassures Dolores that she is "on her side," using a voice that is quietly impassioned so that it expresses her heartfelt concern for Dolores' predicament. Dr. B also makes an effort to connect with her as a woman living in a society with ongoing gender oppression, thinking that Dolores might see that Dr. B understands structural racism by analogy with sexism. Dolores becomes less agitated and moves slightly away from the wall as they continue to talk. Dr. B then asks Dolores how she would explain that Dr. H is concerned about the potential for violence, repeatedly reassuring her that she is open to the possibility that Dolores may be a victim of racism. As she tells her story, Dolores seems to open up somewhat. She cries while appearing angry about events in her current life and becomes more upset as she continues to talk. She then tells Dr. B that she does indeed feel furious enough to hurt someone. Dr. B asks questions to ascertain her intent and degree of planning. Dolores says she does not mean she would "really" hurt someone but that she feels angry enough to do so. After listening, Dr. B explains that she accepts Dolores' perspective that her neighbors are racist toward her but that she also believes that she might be having some mental troubles that make it more difficult for her to cope with stress. Dr. B suggests that Dolores might benefit from a short stay in a hospital where she can feel safe while receiving short-term medication to decrease her stress. Dolores expresses anger and distrust at the suggestion, saying she does not need "incarceration" for something that is other people's fault. Dr. B does not really believe that Dolores is dangerous and wonders to herself whether she has been captive to an old epistemology of ignorance in suggesting that Dolores be hospitalized. Still, she offers anti-anxiety medication to Dolores to help her cope with her stress, along with a follow-up visit. Dolores becomes angry with Dr. B and exclaims that she cannot trust her. Dr. B ends the session while still standing (an awkward arrangement, in her mind), requesting that Dolores make a follow-up appointment to talk more about her recent troubles. Dr. B makes a mental note to talk with her group of colleagues about her session with Dolores before Dolores' next appointment.

Dr. B did many things right: she didn't assume either that Dolores was mentally ill or that she was not; she didn't assume that she, Dr. B, would be viewed as trustworthy or an expert; she tried to empathize with Dolores and to use analogical reasoning to help forge connections between them; she avoided pathologizing Dolores' acts of defiance while leaving open the question that her defiance may be symptomatic; she counted Dolores as a knower with local knowledge of race and gender relations; and she drew upon her understanding of how psychiatric epistemologies of ignorance and resistance work in order to give uptake to Dolores. Perhaps most importantly, Dr. B did not reinforce defiance as a burdened virtue in Dolores. It is possible that Dolores's righteous indignation at racism is a trait v_4 burdened virtue (see Chapter 3). Yet, because Dr. B reconceptualizes defiance as a less-burdened or even unburdened virtue, she is in a position to avoid entrenching burdened virtues that may be at play in Dolores.

Still, it was not an entirely successful session. She might have been holding a stereotype of the loud Latina woman, a stereotype that prevented her from drawing on her clinical background to make a clear assessment of the degree to which mental illness was present or absent. Dr. B made missteps, not necessarily by suggesting hospitalization to Dolores but by not adequately interrogating her own psychiatric *episteme* before suggesting it. Perhaps she should have asked questions about Dolores' family history; perhaps she—like Aristotle's bent wood that needs straightening[6]—went too far in an effort not to conflate responses to racism with mental dysfunction. Maybe she should have tried again to get Dolores and herself situated in chairs.

I have deliberately presented this case as one that illustrates an insightful, critically reflective psychiatrist who is committed to being epistemically and ethically responsible in her practice, giving uptake rightly because it is intrinsically good to give uptake to others and because it facilitates good diagnosis and treatment. An encounter like this, even with its less than ideal outcomes, would take effort and engagement with other similar-minded colleagues to be able to do. But it needs to be an aim, because giving uptake rightly in this rich sense is a virtue that is necessary for good psychiatric practice—and because it is the right thing to do. If psychiatrists do not want—even inadvertently and indirectly—to perpetuate systemic injustices, they will need to exercise critical reflection regarding possible tendencies toward epistemic vices and the potential for character change. Such reflection on epistemic fault lines will enable them to move toward corrective and more complete knowing. Giving uptake properly is one way that clinicians can begin to undo the presumptions of knowing and resistances to knowing while, at the same time, diagnosing and treating people more accurately and helpfully. It also is one way to make more accurate diagnoses and avoid mistaking good defiance for a symptom of mental disorder.

In this chapter, my aim has been to set out my theory of uptake, to analyze how giving uptake is relevant to people who behave defiantly, and to indicate difficulties in giving uptake well—in particular, to defiance. Giving uptake is not applicable in the same ways, or to the same extent, in all settings, for all diagnoses, or for all patients. Some settings are more conducive to giving uptake; for example, in the emergency room or in initial assessment, when a diagnosis might be called for, giving uptake rightly may be especially important to focus on in order to avoid misdiagnosing. Additionally, it might not be appropriate to give uptake in the sense of treating the communicator as credible—for example, when a patient is paranoid or delusional. Even here, though, a patient with a history of paranoia still may accurately report that her husband is being abusive and, so, giving uptake to her communications of fear and concern would be crucial to her safety and her health. Furthermore, because giving uptake is a virtue, with extremes and an intermediate, one might give uptake to a degree without quite finding the mean. Learning to give uptake rightly is dispositional; it takes effort, practice, and support from others in order not to fall into epistemic vices and defensive strategies. It might require psychiatrists to act *as if* they are giving uptake well without being fully on board; acting is part of the process of any virtue becoming a character trait. It is important to note, however, that pretending to give uptake is not itself a virtue, because virtues by definition are part of our internal character and epistemic structure.

6.6 **Conclusion**

Some people suffer from mental distress, and many people suffer from adverse living conditions, including oppression. Psychiatrists can and have helped many people to heal, or at least to manage their distress, but they may not always sufficiently attend to the ways that people's adverse living conditions affect them. I have argued that it is always important to identify areas of vulnerability in one's profession and to understand what is involved in challenging entrenched and invisible problems. As I explained in Chapter 5, such contestations of practices require that we employ what Harding calls "strong objectivity," by which she means that scientific communities need critically to examine their own practices, interests, assumptions, and biases. They need to notice and, often, contest the tools and measures and the attitudes toward their objects of study—in the case of psychiatry, the people or patients themselves (Harding 1993). Because none of us is an infallible knower or invulnerable to errors in belief and reasoning or to unintentionally reproducing structurally damaging practices, a stance of strong objectivity is required by all those who practice psychiatry. Even those psychiatrists who already are critically reflective and do not complacently endorse potentially harmful practices could usefully participate in dialogue with other psychiatrists and with service users: constructive change in practices is a collective endeavor, not an individual one. The scope of those to whom this chapter is addressed, therefore, includes all those whose lives are touched by psychiatry—mental health services, service users, and their loved ones—of all colors, classes, and genders. We learn from each other—including the voices of patients who currently are silenced or misunderstood—about the mistakes in thinking, the assumptions, disagreements, weaknesses, and strengths of our practices. Those psychiatrists who already engage in strong objectivity play an important role in identifying with others the aspects of psychiatry that need to be changed in order better to provide care to all service users. Strong objectivity is relevant especially when psychiatrists are working with people who are, or who seem to be, exhibiting defiant behavior; strong objectivity is necessary in order to give uptake rightly.

Therapeutically, when psychiatrists give uptake rightly, they open up the possibility that the patient can strengthen virtues (both intellectual and character ones) and diminish vices. I am not suggesting that psychiatry is in the work of moral redemption, but that a richer understanding of epistemic pitfalls, and virtues such as defiance and uptake, can facilitate patients' insights into their own moral damage due to social structures. This is especially important to those whose virtues are burdened. That is, dialogical responsiveness to people whose social disadvantages and adverse living conditions position them to develop burdened character traits enables them, over time, to lighten those burdened virtues.

Strong objectivity makes it possible for patients as well as psychiatrists to alter patterns of behavior and of thought. Nevertheless, as Code points out, "The persistence of intransigent gender, racial, class-, and ethnicity-based stereotypes, among others embedded in the everyday visible and verbal imagery of science and expertise, is just one reminder of how much remains to be done" (Code 2006, 266). The work of cultivating intellectual and ethical virtues is ongoing and, as I stated in the Introduction, is not done by following principles but, instead, by learning to find the mean, which mean cannot be identified in advance of the context of situated knowers and local practices. This conclusion may be unsatisfactory in that it does not provide concrete guidance that readers can follow, but that is the reality of ethical life: the specificity of what it means to be good is up to us to work through.

Notes

Introduction

1. Medicalization is a process in which human problems become constructed as medical ones (Sadler et al. 2009). An example of medicalization would be to diagnose anxiety and depression about being out of work and out of money as clinical depression. See Porter (2015) for a critical analysis of diagnosing depression.

2. Kleinman refers both to the mistake of imposing diagnostic criteria from one culture onto another and to the mistake of reifying socially caused human suffering into psychiatric problems.

3. By "Othering" I mean the process of marking and naming those whom we see as different from ourselves in ways we take to be significant; they magnify and reinforce projections of ourselves that we consciously or unconsciously reject and tend to reproduce patterns of domination and subordination (Johnson et al. 2004, 254).

Chapter 1

1. Communication with Deborah Spitz, M.D.

2. Communication with Deborah Spitz, M.D.

3. Discussion with Robert Kruger, M.D. Most, but not all of this section on child psychiatry, is informed by personal communication with Dr. Kruger.

4. Communication with Marilyn Frye, 2015.

5. Note I disagree that accountability signifies correlative rights, but I do not defend this here.

Chapter 2

1. See also Andrew Scull (1983) for an historical account of the domestication of madness.

2. This is a composite case drawn from my experiences of attending emergency psychiatric services.

Chapter 4

1. Lawrence Pervin gives a good critical analysis of the underlying assumptions in trait theory (Pervin 1994).

2. Neuroscientific studies also indicate differences in neural structures that might explain different subtypes of CD (Frick et al. 2014; Jones et al. 2009).

3. It is a curious finding that aggression, regardless of gender, does not elicit victim empathy even when the aggressor is not judged to be justified. Other studies suggest that even toddlers seem to have victim empathy (see Hamlin et al. 2011) but to try to fill in this gap would take me too far afield.

4. I owe this way of explaining the difficulty in determining the facts about social aggression to John Sadler.

5. See www.slutwalktoronto.com.

6. Children's ideas of harm and help do not arise naturally: they already are socialized into stereotype formation and their accounts of harms may reflect this. Furthermore, as we teach our children (construing the term "our children" broadly here) how to treat others, what actions are hurtful and why, and, in general, to habituate them well into avoiding harmful behavior, many adults assume they know what is right and wrong. (Others are wracked with ambivalence and uncertainty.) We, too, though, are socialized within structures of advantage and disadvantage and have formed habits of thought and beliefs about values, worth, and fairness. Our ideas about good and bad behavior, and what should be done about it, vary not only with local customs and communities, but also with our particular situatedness with respect to privileges and privations.

7. I have argued elsewhere (Potter 2014) that racial stereotypes of Black males in interpreting their behavior as defiant may lead to a misdiagnosis of ODD and that such biases may suffuse the classification itself. That argument would extend this chapter beyond necessity: here I focus on the complex matrices of childhood development and ways to understand defiance in those contexts.

8. As an example of norms for whiteliness I offer a family experience from one of our daughters' high school graduations. Her school was a primarily white school and, at the graduation, the master of ceremonies warned that there was to be no standing applause and cheering of graduates—that we were to sit circumspectly and hold our applause until all had received their diplomas. But that edict went against the style of the local African American families, and so they defied the edict to behave "civilly" according to white norms. They were routinely removed from the auditorium by police, on the grounds that they were disruptive. Deviations from whitely norms are not tolerated; the conflict between norms is resolved not by weighing the value of one set of norms over the other but by the megaphone, police backing, and authority of a majority of the white community.

9. I make a strong claim by saying it is "always" produced in these ways, but even a neurologically based aggression occurs within an external environment. Aggression in children can be biologically triggered or not, depending on factors we do not yet understand.

10. The researchers did not identify the ethnicity of specific participants whose voices appeared in their paper.

11. In their study of adolescent girls, they found that many girls believed that girls' friendships were quite fragile, such that they had to be vigilant in maintaining them. They used threat exclusions and other strategies to gain power and avoid abandonment. These researchers' findings suggest that norms of femininity restrict the available options to girls for conflict management (Crothers, Field, and Kolbert 2005).

12. Rights-talk is individualistic; it frames the needs of people in terms of their ontological and social status as individuals. In this book, I move away from a strictly individualist way of thinking about what it means to be a person. I believe that we are always embedded in discursively produced historical, social, and legal positions and that to extract us from those contexts is artifactual and a way of reproducing and justifying inequalities. But I do not argue for this position.

Chapter 5

1. Considerable debate exists about the relationship between psychopathy and antisociality, but this debate will not be taken up (see the work of Skeem and Cooke 2010; Oglaff 2006). Oglaff argues that the two are conflated, with the result that far too many people qualify for a diagnosis of ASPD than is warranted (Oglaff 2010, 521).

2. Although a theory of legal harms and norms might be helpful, I cannot provide one here. See Joel Feinberg (1990).

3. I owe this qualification, the wording, and examples to Lisa Tessman.

4. In philosophical terms, I am not a strict internalist, although I find internalism appealing. But an understanding of the internalism/externalism debates on knowing are unnecessary for this book.

5. Aristotle distinguishes between theoretical reasoning, which involves those things that "do not admit of being otherwise, such as mathematics and scientific knowledge." See Aristotle (1999, Bk. VI).

6. For example, Rawls' constructivist account of the principles of justice fails, on O'Neill's view, because he imports idealized assumptions about human reasoning that he does not justify.

7. Peterson thinks that a concept of harm from counterfactual baselines is a more plausible account than other contenders. On his view, an individual is harmed by another individual (or a group of individuals) if and only if the latter person, either by doing or allowing an act, brings it about that the former individual is worse off in terms of well-being than she or he would have been in the absence of that act (Peterson 2014, 102). I resist going in the direction of counterfactuals for two reasons. One is that counterfactuals rely on possible worlds, and my interest is in *this* world. Secondly, I think some harms are non-comparative.

8. Morton proposes that

   > we should think of the norms of rationality ecologically: that is, the norms that constitute rational practical deliberation depend on the complex interaction between the psychological capacities of the agent in question and the agent's environment. If we think of the norms of practical deliberation ecologically, a complex picture emerges of the kind of justification we can offer for particular norms of practical deliberation; most importantly, that justification will have to be sensitive to empirical considerations. (Morton 2010, 561–2)

   The ecological context interacts with norms of deliberation. The complexity of environmental considerations in practical deliberation is made even more complex by the deliberative person's psychology. Norms of reasoning need to account for a person's psychology—for example, a person might tend to discount the future or be biased toward purely self-centered goals. So, we need norms governing how and when we should discount the future, when and to what extent we should disregard the needs of others, and how to prioritize our various desires. Finally, a general account of practical deliberation says that, if some action is good, then one has a reason to perform that action. But given people's (varying) tendencies to discount or to fail to consider whole classes of considerations due to biases and stereotypes, and our propensity toward self-deception, we need a norm for those who have trouble identifying what is good in a given context.

9. Recent neurocognitive research by Blair, Mitchell, and Blair (2005) locates moral impairments in a dysfunction of the amygdala. In earlier work, Blair (1995) proposed a model of a violence inhibition mechanism (VIM) that is necessary for the development of moral emotions (sympathy, guilt, remorse, and empathy), and the inhibiting of one's violent behavior. He argues that VIM is necessary for the development of moral emotions and hypothesizes that the absence of a functioning VIM can explain the development of psychopathology (Blair 1995).

10. For more on the recovery movement, see Davidson, Rakfeldt, and Strauss (2011).

11. I have phrased Henry's defiance as "in the direction of praiseworthy" but, because it is unclear as yet what level of functioning Henry will be able to achieve given his diagnosis, it may only ever be "in the direction of." It is an open question whether Henry's defiance could meet the condition of Tessman's trait v_1 where choices and actions are partly constitutive of a flourishing life. It may be that Henry's defiance best fits trait v_2.

Chapter 6

1. See Potter 2000 and Potter 2009, ch. 5, for other discussions of this virtue.

2. Granted, Austin did not intend his concept of uptake to go beyond the constraints he employs. I think his concept is important enough that it should be used more widely, but that requires extending it.

3. Avery Kolers, personal communication 2015.

4. Mona Gupta, personal communication 2015.

5. Some of these points are drawn from Potter (2015).

6. Aristotle NE 1999, 1109b1–8.

References

Alcoff, Linda. 2007. Epistemologies of ignorance: Three types. In *Race and epistemologies of ignorance*, eds. S. Sullivan and N. Tuana, 39–57. Albany, NY: State University of New York Press.

Alexander, Michelle. 2012. *The new Jim Crow: Mass incarceration in the age of colorblindness*. New York: The New Press.

Allison, Dorothy. 1993. *Bastard out of Carolina*. New York: Plume.

American Psychiatric Association. 1994. *Diagnostic and statistical manual of mental disorder*, 4th edn. Arlington, VA: American Psychiatric Publishing.

American Psychiatric Association. 2000. *Diagnostic and statistical manual of mental disorder*, 4th edn. text revision. Arlington, VA: American Psychiatric Publishing.

American Psychiatric Association. 2013. *Diagnostic and statistical manual of mental disorders*, 5th edn. Arlington, VA: American Psychiatric Publishing.

American Psychiatric Association Work Group on Eating Disorders. 2000. Practice guideline for the treatment of patients with eating disorders (revision). *American Journal of Psychiatry* **157** (1 Suppl):1–39

Aristotle.1985. *Nicomachean ethics*. trans. Terence Irwin. Indianapolis: Hackett Pub. Co.

Aristotle. 2000. *Nichomachean ethics*. 2nd edn. trans. Terence Irwin. Hackett Pub. Co.

Aronson, Jeffrey. 2007. Compliance, concordance, adherence. *British Journal of Clinical Pharmacology* **63** (4):383–4.

Austin, J.L. 1975. *How to do things with words*, ed. J.O. Urmson and M. Sbisa. Cambridge, MA: Harvard University Press.

Babiak, Paul, Craig Neumann, and Robert Hare. 2010. Corporate psychopathy: Talking the walk. *Behavioral Sciences and the Law* **28**:174–93.

Baier, Annette. 1985. *Postures of the mind: Essays on mind and morals*. Minneapolis: University of Minnesota Press.

Baier, Annette. 2004. Demoralization, trust, and the virtues. In *Setting the moral compass: Essays by women philosophers*, ed. C. Calhoun, 176–88. Oxford: Oxford University Press.

Bailey, Alison. 2007. Strategic ignorance. In *Race and epistemologies of ignorance*, eds. S. Sullivan and N. Tuana, 77–94. Albany, NY: State University of New York Press.

Bandura, A. 1986. Social foundations of thought and action: A social cognitive theory. Englewood Cliffs, NJ: Prentice Hall.

Berkel, Cady, Velma McBride Murry, Tera R. Hurt, and Yi-fu Chen. 2009. It takes a village: Protecting rural African American youth in the context of racism. *Journal of Youth and Adolescence* **38** (2):175–88.

Best, Stephen. 1995. *The politics of historical vision: Marx, Foucault, Habermas*. New York: Guilford Press.

Blair, James. 1995. A cognitive developmental approach to morality: Investigating the psychopath. *Cognition* **57**(1):1–29.

Blair, James. 2013. The neurobiology of psychopathic traits in youths. *Nature Reviews Neuroscience* **14** (11):786–99.

Blair, James, Ellen Leibenluft, and Daniel Pine. 2014. Conduct disorder and callous-unemotional traits in youth. *New England Journal of Medicine* **371** (23):2207–16.

Blair, James, Derek Mitchell, and Karina Blair. 2005. *The psychopath: Emotion and the brain*. Malden, MA: Blackwell Publishing.

Block, Sidney, and Stephen Green. *Psychiatric ethics*, 4th edn. Oxford: Oxford University Press.

Blum, Lawrence. 2004. Stereotypes and stereotyping: A moral analysis. *Philosophical Papers* **33**(3): 251–89.

Bosak, Janine, Sabine Sczesny, and Alice Eagly. 2012. The impact of social roles on trait judgments: A critical reexamination. *Personality and Social Psychology Bulletin* **38** (4):429–40.

Boxill, Bernard. 1995. Self-respect and protest. In *Dignity, character, and self-respect*, ed. R. Dillon, 93–104. London and New York: Routledge.

Brehm, Sharon and Jack Brehm. 2013. *Psychological reactance: A theory of freedom and control*. London: Academic Press.

Brennan, Geoffrey, Lina Eriksson, Robert E. Goodin, and Nicholas Southwood. 2013. *Explaining norms*. Oxford: Oxford University Press.

Brody, G.H., Y.F. Chen, and V. M. Murry, et al. 2006. Perceived discrimination and the adjustment of African American youths: A five-year longitudinal analysis with contextual moderation effects. *Child Development* **77** (5):1170–89.

Cadet, Danielle. 2013. Black boys considered "cool" and "tough" while Black girls stereotyped as "ghetto" and "loud" in suburban schools, October 30, 2013. *The Huffington Post*. TheHuffintonPost.com, Inc. http://www.huffingtonpost.com/2013/10/22/black-boys-in-school-black-girls_n_4151328.html. Last accessed January 14, 2015.

Calhoun, Cheshire. 2004. Common decency. In *Setting the moral compass: Essays by women philosophers*, ed. C. Calhoun, 128–42. Oxford: Oxford University Press.

Card, Claudia. 1990. Gender and moral luck. In *Identity, character, morality: Essays in moral psychology*, ed. O. Flanagan and A. Rorty, 199–218. Cambridge: MIT Press.

Card, Claudia. 1996. *The unnatural lottery: Character and moral luck*. Philadelphia: Temple University Press.

Card, Claudia. 2005. *The atrocity paradigm: A theory of evil*. Oxford: Oxford University Press.

Cartwright, Samuel. 2004. Report on the diseases and physical peculiarities of the Negro race. In *Health, disease, and illness: Concepts in medicine*, ed. Arthur Caplan, McCartney James, and Sisti Dominic, 28–39. Washington, D.C.: Georgetown University Press.

Caygill, Howard. 2013. *On resistance: A philosophy of defiance*. New York: Bloomsbury.

Centorrino, Franca, Miguel Hernán, Giuseppa Drago-Ferrante, Melanie Rendall, et al. 2001. Factors associated with noncompliance with psychiatric outpatient visits. *Psychiatric Services* **52** (3):378–80.

Cheng, Nien.1987. *Life and death in Shanghai*. New York: Penguin Books.

Chida, Y. and **A. Steptoe**. 2008. Positive psychological well-being and mortality: A quantitative review of prospective observational studies. *Psychosomatic Medicine* **70** (7):741–56.

Cockburn, Henry and **Patrick Cockburn**. 2011. *Henry's demons: Living with schizophrenia, a father and son's story.* New York: Scribner.

Code, Lorraine. 1991. *What can she know? Feminist theory and the construction of knowledge.* Ithaca: Cornell University Press.

Code, Lorraine. 2006. *Ecological thinking: The politics of epistemic location.* Oxford: Oxford University Press.

Code, Lorraine. 2008. Advocacy, negotiation, and the politics of unknowing. *The Southern Journal of Philosophy* **Vol XLVI**: 32–51.

Coker, T.R., M.N. Elliott, D.E. Kanouse, J.A. Grunbaum, et al. 2009. Perceived racial/ethnic discrimination among fifth-grade students and its association with mental health. *American Journal of Public Health* **99** (5):878–84

Collins, Patricia. 1990. *Black feminist thought: Knowledge, consciousness, and the politics of empowerment.* New York: Routledge.

Coplan, Amy. 2011. Understanding empathy: Its features and effects. In *Empathy: Philosophical and psychological perspectives*, 3–18. Oxford: Oxford University Press.

Coyne, Sarah M., John Archer, Mike Eslea, and **Toni Liechty**. 2008. Adolescent perceptions of indirect forms of relational aggression: Sex of perpetrator effects. *Aggressive Behavior* **34** (6), 577–83.

Crenshaw, Kimberlé. 1991. Mapping the margins: Intersectionality, identity politics, and violence against women of color. *Stanford Law Review* **43** (6): 1241–99.

Crick, Nicki. 1997. Engagement in gender normative versus nonnormative forms of aggression: Links to social–psychological adjustment. *Developmental Psychology* **33** (4):610–7.

Crick, Nickki, Jamie Ostrov, Karen Appleyard, Elizabeth A. Jansen, and Juan F. Casas. 2004. Relational aggression in early childhood: "You can't come to my birthday party unless …". In *Aggression, antisocial behavior, and violence among girls: A developmental perspective*, ed. M. Putallaz and K. Bierman, 71–89. New York: Guilford Press.

Crittendon, P.M., and **M.D.S. Ainsworth**. 1989. Child maltreatment and attachment theory. In *Child maltreatment: Theories and research on the causes and consequences of child abuse and neglect*, ed. D. Cicchetti and V. Carlson, 432–63. Cambridge: Cambridge University Press.

Croskerry, Pat. 2009. Clinical cognition and diagnostic error: Applications of a dual process model of reasoning. *Advances in Health Science Education* **14** (S1):27–35.

Crothers, Laura, Julaine Field, and **Jered Kolbert**. 2005. Navigating power, control, and being nice: Aggression in adolescent girls' friendships. *Journal of Counseling and Development* **83** (3): 349–54.

Crowe, S.L., and **B. Blair**. 2008. The development of antisocial behavior: What can we learn from functional neuroimagining studies? *Development and Psychopathology* **20** (4):1145–59.

Cuomo, Chris J. 1998. *Feminism and ecological communities: An ethic of flourishing.* New York: Routledge.

Currie, Dawn, Deirdre Kelly, and Shauna Pomerantz. 2007. "The power to squash people": Understanding girls' relational aggression. *British Journal of Sociology of Education* **28** (1):23–37.

Dahl, Norman. 1984. *Practical reason, Aristotle, and weakness of the will*. Minneapolis, MN: University of Minnesota Press.

Dan-Cohen, Meir. 1994. In defense of defiance. *Philosophy and Public Affairs* 23(1): 24–51.

Davidson, Larry, Jaak Rakfeldt, and John Strauss. 2011. *The roots of the recovery movement in psychiatry: Lessons learned*. Chichester, UK: Wiley-Blackwell.

Deigh, John. 2014. Psychopathic resentment. In *Being amoral: Psychopathy and moral incapacity*, ed. Thomas Schramme, 209–26. Cambridge, MA: The MIT Press.

Denn, Rebekah. 2002. Blacks are disciplined at far higher rates than other students. In *Seattle Post-intelligencer*, March 14, 2002.

Dias, Karen. 2003. The Ana sanctuary: Women's pro-anorexia narratives in cyberspace. *Journal of International Women's Studies* 4 (2):31–45.

Diener, E., J.F. Helliwell, and D. Kahneman. 2010. *International differences in well-being*. New York: Oxford University Press.

Ditrich, Hans. 2015. Cognitive fallacies and criminal investigations. *Science and Justice* 55 (2):155–9.

Dolan, P., T. Peasgood, and M.P. White. 2008. Do we really know what makes us happy? A review of the economic literature on the factors associated with subjective well-being. *Journal of Economic Psychology* **29**: 94–122.

Dostoevsky, Fyodor. 1960. *Notes from underground: And the grand inquisitor*. New York: Dutton.

Doza, Christine. 2001. Bloodlove. In *Listen up! Voices from the next feminist generation*, ed. B. Findlen, 40–7. Emeryville, CA: Seal Press.

Draper, Heather. 2000. Anorexia nervosa and respecting a refusal of life-prolonging therapy: A limited justification. *Bioethics* 14 (2):120–33.

Endler, Norman S. and Nancy Kocovski. 2001. State and trait anxiety revisited. *Journal of Anxiety Disorders* 15 (3):231–45.

Espeset, E.M., R.H. Nordbo, K.S. Gulliksen, F. Skårderud, et al. 2011. The concept of body image disturbance in anorexia nervosa: An empirical inquiry utilizing patients' subjective experiences. *Eating Disorders* 19 (2):175–93.

Fadiman, Anne. 1997. *The spirit catches you and you fall down*. New York: Farrar, Straus and Giroux.

Falcón y Tella, María. 2004. Civil disobedience and test cases. *Ratio Juris* 17(3): 315–27.

Fanon, Franz. 2008. *Black skin, white masks*, trans. R. Philcox. New York: Grove Press.

Farrelly, Simone, Helen Lester, Diana Rose, Max Birchwood, et al. 2015. Barriers to shared decision making in mental health care: Qualitative study of the Joint Crisis Plan for psychosis. *Health Expectations*, early view April 27 2015. doi: 10.1111/hex.12368

Feinberg, Joel. 1990. *Harmless wrongdoing: The moral limits of the criminal law*. Oxford: Oxford University Press.

Ferguson, Ann A. 2001. *Bad boys: Public schools in the making of Black masculinity*. Ann Arbor, MI: University of Michigan Press.

Fernandez, Manny and Erik Eckholm. 2014. "Pregnant, and forced to stay on life support." *New York Times*, January 8, 2014. http://www.nytimes.com/2014/01/08/us/pregnant-and-forced-to-stay-on-life-support.html?_r=0. Last accessed May 8, 2015.

Fernando, Suman. 2012. Race and culture issues in mental health and some thoughts on ethnic identity. *Counselling Psychology Quarterly* 25 (2):113–23.

Finley, Laurene. 1997. The multiple effects of culture and ethnicity on psychiatric disability. In *Psychological and social aspects of psychiatric disability*, ed. LeRoy Spaniol, Cheryl Gagne, and Martin Koehler, 497–510. Boston, MA: Center for Psychiatric Rehabilitation.

Fogarty, Jeanne S., and George A. Youngs. 2000. Psychological reactance as a factor in patient noncompliance with medication taking: A field experiment. *Journal of Applied Social Psychology* 30 (11):2365–91.

Fox, Nick, Katie Ward, and Alan O'Rourke. 2005. Pro-anorexia, weight-loss drugs and the internet: An "anti-recovery" explanatory model of anorexia. *Sociology of Health & Illness* 27 (7):944–71.

Frese, Frederick J., Edward L. Knight, and Elyn Saks. 2009. Recovery from schizophrenia: With views of psychiatrists, psychologists, and others diagnosed with this disorder. *Schizophrenia Bulletin* 35 (2):370–80.

Freud, Sigmund. 2005. *Civilization and its discontents*. New York: WW Norton and Co.

Frick, P.J. 2006. Developemental pathways to conduct disorder. *Child and Adolescent Psychiatric Clinics of North America* 15 (2):311–31.

Frick, P. J., and M. Ellis. 1999. Callous-unemotional traits and subtypes of conduct disorder. *Clinical Child and Family Psychology Review* 2 (3):149–68.

Frick, P.J., J.V. Ray, L.C. Thornton, and R.E. Kahn. 2014a. Can callous-unemotional traits enhance the understanding, diagnosis, and treatment of serious conduct problems in children and adolescents? A comprehensive review. *Psychological Bulletin* 140 (1):1–57.

Frick, P.J., J.V. Ray, L.C. Thornton, and R.E. Kahn. 2014b. Annual research review: A developmental psychopathology approach to understanding callous-unemotional traits in children and adolescents with serious conduct problems. *Journal of Child Psychology and Psychiatry* 55 (6):532–48.

Fricker, Miranda. 2007. *Epistemic Injustice: Power and the ethics of knowing*. Oxford: Oxford University Press.

Frosch, Dominick L., Suepattra G. May, Katherine A.S. Rendle, Caroline Tietbohl, et al. 2012. Authoritarian physicians and patients' fear of being "difficult" among key obstacles to shared decision-making. *Health Affairs* 31 (5):1030–8.

Frye, Marilyn. 1983. *The politics of reality: Essays in feminist theory*. Freedom, CA: Crossing Press.

Frye, Marilyn. 1992. White woman feminist. In *Willful virgin: Essays in feminism 1976–1992*. Berkeley, CA: Crossing Press.

Furth, Montgomery. 1988. *Substance, form, and psyche: An Aristotelian metaphysics*. Cambridge, MA: Cambridge University Press.

Gammelgaard, Judith. 2003. Ego, self, and otherness. *Scandinavian Psychoanalytic Review* 26:96–108.

Garety, Philippa A., and David R. Hemsley. 1994. *Delusions: Investigations into the psychology of delusional reasoning*. New York and Oxford: Oxford University Press.

Garrett, Barbara, and Tom Posey. 1997. Involuntary commitment: A consumer perspective. In *Psychological and Social Aspects of Psychiatric Disability*, ed. L. Spaniol, C. Gagne, and M. Koehler, 503–6. Center for Psychiatric Rehabilitation: Boston University.

Gee, James, Glynda Hull, and Colin Lankshear. 1996. *The new work order.* Sydney, Australia: Allen and Unwin.

Gert, Bernard, and Timothy Duggan. 1979. Free will as the ability to will. *Nous* **13** (2):197–217.

Gilligan, Carol, and Lynn Brown. 1992. *Meeting at the crossroads: Women's psychology and girls' development.* Cambridge, Mass: Harvard University Press.

Gilman, Sander. 1985. *Difference and pathology: Stereotypes of sexuality, race, and madness.* Ithaca, NY: Cornell University Press.

Gladwell, Malcolm. 2007. *Blink: The power of thinking without thinking.* New York: Little, Brown and Company.

Goldfarb, Jeffrey. 1998. *Civility and subversion: The intellectual in democratic society.* Cambridge: Cambridge University Press.

Goldie, Peter. 2000. *The emotions: A philosophical exploration.* Oxford: Clarendon Press.

Gone, J.P. 2008. "So I can be like a whiteman": The cultural psychology of space and place in American Indian mental health. *Culture and Psychology* **14** (3):369–99.

Goodin, Robert. 1985. *Protecting the vulnerable.* Chicago: University of Chicago Press.

Hacking, Ian. 1999. *The social construction of what?* Cambridge, MA: Harvard University Press.

Haidt, Jonathan. 2001. The emotional dog and its rational tail: A social intuitionist approach to moral judgment. *Psychological Review* **108** (4):814–34.

Hale, J. 2009. Tracing a ghostly memory in my throat: Reflections on FtM feminist voice and agency. In *You've changed: Sex reassignment and personal identity*, ed. L. J. Shrage, 43–65. Oxford: Oxford University Press.

Halpern, Jodi. 2001. *From detached concern to empathy: Humanizing medical practice.* Oxford: Oxford University Press.

Hamann, J., S. Leucht, and W. Kissing. 2003. Shared decision making in psychiatry. *Acta Psychiatrica Scandinavica* **107** (6):403–9.

Hamlin, J. Kiley, Karen Wynn, Paul Bloom, and Neha Mahajan. 2001. How infants and toddlers react to antisocial others. *Proceedings of the National Academy of Sciences* **108** (50):19931–6.

Haraway, Donna. 1988. Situated knowledges: The science question in feminism and the privilege of partial perspective. *Feminist Studies* **1** (3): 575–99.

Harding, Sandra. 1993. Rethinking standpoint epistemology: What is "strong objectivity"? *Feminist Epistemologies*, ed. Linda Alcoff and Elizabeth Potter, 49–82. New York: Routledge.

Hare, Robert. 2001. Psychopathy and risk for recidivism and violence. In *Criminal Justice Mental Health and the Politics of Risk*, ed. Nicola S. Gray, Judith M. Laing, and Leslie Noaks, 27–48. New York: Routledge.

Hare, Robert, and Craig S. Neumann. 2009. Psychopathy: Assessment and forensic implications. *Canadian Journal of Psychiatry* **54** (12):791–802.

Harrosh, Shlomit. 2011. Identifying harms. *Bioethics* **26** (9):493–8.

Hartmann, Heinz. 1964. Comments on the psychoanalytic theory of the ego. In *Essays on ego psychology: Selected problems in psychoanalytic theory*. New York: International Universities Press.

Haslanger, Sally. 2014. Social meaning and philosophical method. *Proceedings and Addresses of the American Philosophical Association* **88**: 16–37.

Hedges, Chris, and Joe Sacco. 2012. *Days of destruction, days of revolt*. New York: Nation Books.

Herman, Barbara. 2004. The scope of moral requirement. In *Setting the moral compass: Essays by women philosophers*, ed. C. Calhoun, 91–112. Oxford: Oxford University Press.

Hesse-Biber, Sharlene Nagy. 2006. *The Cult of Thinness*, 2nd edn., Oxford: Oxford University Press.

Hill, Thomas. 1995. Servility and self-respect. In *Dignity, character, and self-respect*, ed. R. Dillon, 76–92. London and New York: Routledge.

Hines, Paulette M., and Nancy Boyd-Franklin. 1996. African American families. *In Ethnicity and family therapy*, ed. M. McGoldrick, J. Giordano, and J. Pearce, 87–100. New York: Guilford Press.

The Hub Staff Report. 2014. "JHU Ethicist considers case of pregnant woman forced to stay on life support." *John Hopkins University News Network*, January 9, 2014. http://hub.jhu.edu/2014/01/09/texas-woman-life-support-pregnancy. Last accessed May 27, 2014

Hubbard, Julie A. 2001. Emotion expression processes in children's peer interaction: The role of peer rejection, aggression, and gender. *Child Development* **72** (5):1426–38.

Hume, David. 1975. *A treatise of human nature*, 2nd edn., eds. L. A. Selby-Bigge and P. H. Nidditch. Oxford: Clarendon Press.

Huppert, Felicia. 2009. Psychological well-being: Evidence regarding its causes and consequences. *Applied Psychology: Health and Well-being* **1** (2):137–64.

Huppert, Felicia and Timothy So. 2013. Flourishing across Europe: Application of a new conceptual framework for defining well-being. *Social Indicators Research* **110** (3):837–61.

Hursthouse, Rosalind. 1996. Normative virtue ethics. In *How should one live? Essays on the Virtues*, ed. Roger Crisp, 19–36. Oxford: Oxford University Press.

Ipsa-Landa, Simone. 2013. Gender, race, and justifications for group exclusion: Urban Black students bussed to affluent suburban schools. *Sociology of Education* **86** (3):218–33.

Jadad, Alejandro R., Carlos A. Rizo, and Murray W. Enkin. 2003. I am a good patient, believe it or not. *British Medical Journal* **326** (7402):1293–5.

Jaggar, Alison. 1989. Love and knowledge: Emotion in feminist epistemology. *Inquiry: An Interdisciplinary Journal of Philosophy* **32** (2):151–76.

Johnson, Joy, Joan Bottoroff, Annette Brown, et al. 2004. Othering and being othered in the context of health care services. *Health Communication* **16** (2):253–71.

Jones, Alice P., Kristen R. Laurens, Catherine M. Herba, Gareth J. Barker, and Essi Viding. 2009. Amygdala hypoactivity to fearful faces in boys with conduct problems and callous-unemotional traits. *American Journal of Psychiatry* **166**(1): 95–102

Jones, Nikki. 2009a. "I was aggressive for the streets, pretty for the pictures": Gender, difference, and the inner-city girl. *Gender and Society* **23** (1): 89–93.

Jones, Nikki. 2009b. *Between good and ghetto: African American girls and inner-city violence.* Chapel Hill, NC: Rutgers University Press.

Kaden, M. 2009. *African American adolescent males and conduct disorder: An examination of diagnosis and racial bias.* Dissertation, California Institute of Integral Studies, San Francisco.

Kaliuzhna, Mariia, Valérian Chambon, Nicolas Franck, Bérangère Testud, et al. 2012. Belief revision and delusions: How do patients with schizophrenia take advice? *PLoS ONE* 7 (4):e34771.

Keenan, Kate, and Daniel S. Shaw. 1994. The development of aggression in toddlers: A study of low-income families. *Journal of Abnormal Child Psychology* 22 (1):53–77.

Keyes, Corey and Jonathan Haidt. 2003. *Flourishing: Positive psychology and the life well-lived.* Arlington, VA: American Psychological Association.

Keyes, Corey. 2006. Mental health in adolescence: Is America's youth flourishing? *American Journal of Orthopsychiatry* 76 (3):395–402.

Keyes, Corey. 2007. Promoting and protecting mental health as flourishing: A complementary strategy for improving national mental health. *American Psychologist* 62 (2).95–108.

Keyes, Corey. 2009. The Black–White paradox in health: Flourishing in the face of social inequality and discrimination. *Journal of Personality* 77 (6):1677–705.

Kleinman, Arthur. 1988. *Rethinking psychiatry: From cultural category to personal experience.* New York: Free Press.

Kleinsinger, Fred. 2010. Working with the noncompliant patient. *The Permanente Journal* 14 (1):54–60.

Kohut, Heinz. 1971. *The analysis of the self: A systematic approach to the psychoanalytic treatment of narcissistic personality disorders.* Madison, CT: International Universities Press.

Kroll, J., A. Yusuf, and K. Fujiwara. 2010. Psychoses, PTSD, and depression in Somali refugees in Minnesota. *Social Psychiatry and Psychiatric Epidemiology* 46 (6):481–93.

Lee, Sing. 2001. Fat phobia in anorexia nervosa: Whose obsession is it? In *Eating Disorders and Cultures in Transition*, ed. M. Nasser, M. A. Katzman, and R. A. Gordon, 37–59. New York: Taylor & Francis Inc.

Lefkowitz, David. 2007. On a moral right to civil disobedience. *Ethics* 117: 202–33.

Lei, Joy. 2003. (Un)necessary toughness?: Those "loud Black girls" and those "quiet Asian boys." *Anthropology and Education Quarterly* 34 (2):158–81.

Lewin, Tamar. 2012. Black students punished more, data suggests. *New York Times*, March 6, 2012.

Linehan, Marcia. 1993. *Cognitive-behavioral treatment of Borderline Personality Disorder.* New York: Guilford Press.

Loeber, R., J. Burke, B. Lahey, A. Winders, and M. Zera. 2000. Oppositional defiant and conduct disorder: A review of the past 10 years, part I. *Journal of the American Academy of Child and Adolescent Psychiatry* 39 (12): 1468–84.

Lugones, María. 2007. Heterosexualism and the Colonial/Modern Gender System. *Hypatia* 22 (1): 186–209.

Lugones, María, and Elizabeth Spelman. 1983. Have we got a theory for you! Feminist theory, cultural imperialism and the demand for "the woman's voice." *Women's Studies International Forum* 6 (6):573–81.

Lyubomirsky, Sonja, Laura King, and **Ed Diener**. 2005. The benefits of frequent positive affect: Does happiness lead to success? *Psychological Bulletin* **131**(6): 803–55.

Mack, John. 1997. Power, powerlessness, and empowerment in psychotherapy. In *Psychological and social aspects of psychiatric disability*, ed. L. Spaniol, C. Gagne, and M. Koehler, 562–84. Center for Psychiatric Rehabilitation: Boston University.

Macsween, Morag. 1993. *Anorexic bodies: A feminist and sociological perspective on Anorexia Nervosa*. London and New York: Routledge.

Martin, Norah. 2001. Feminist bioethics and psychiatry. *Journal of Medicine and Philosophy* **26** (4):431–41.

McCarthy, Alexandra, R. Shaban, J. Boys, and **S. Winch**. 2010. Compliance, normality, and the patient on peritoneal dialysis. *Nephrology Nursing Journal* **37** (3):243–50.

McEachern, Amber D., and **James Snyder**. 2012. Gender differences in predicting antisocial behaviors: Developmental consequences of physical and relational aggression. *Journal of Abnormal Child Psychology* **40** (4):501–12.

McFall, Lynne. 1987. Integrity. *Ethics* **98** (1):5–20.

McGregor, Joan. 2004. Civility, civic virtue, and citizenship. In *Civility and its discontents: Essays on civic virtue, toleration, and cultural fragmentation*, ed. C. T. Sistare, 25–42 Lawrence, Kansas: University of Kansas Press.

McIntosh, Peggy. 1988. White privilege and male privilege: A personal account of coming to see correspondences through work in Women's Studies. Working paper #189. Wellesley, MA: Wellesley College Center for Research on Women.

Medina, José. 2013. *The epistemology of resistance: Gender and racial oppression, epistemic injustice, and resistant imaginations*. Oxford: Oxford University Press.

Megone, Christopher. 2000. Mental illness, human function, and values. *Philosophy, Psychiatry, and Psychology* **7** (1):45–67.

Mele, A.R. 2005. Libertarianism, luck, and control. *Pacific Philosophical Quarterly* **86** (3):381–407.

Mendel, R., E. Traut-Mattausch, E. Jonas, S. Leucht, J. M. Kane, et al. 2011. Confirmation bias: Why psychiatrists stick to wrong preliminary diagnoses. *Psychological Medicine* **41** (12):2651–9.

Metzl, Jonathan. 2009. *The protest psychosis: How schizophrenia became a Black disease*. Boston, MA: Beacon Press.

Mills, Charles. 2007. White ignorance. In *Race and epistemologies of ignorance*, eds. S. Sullivan and N. Tuana, 13–28. Albany, NY: State University of New York Press.

Mills, Charles. 2010. Blacks and social justice: A quarter-century later. *Journal of Social Philosophy* **41** (3):354–69.

Mitchell, Stephen and **Margaret Black**. 1995. *Freud and beyond: A history of modern psychoanalytic thought*. New York: Basic Books.

Moody-Adams, Michele. 1994. Culture, responsibility, and affected ignorance. *Ethics* **104** (2):291–309.

Morgan, Kathryn Pauly. 2011. Foucault, ugly ducklings, and technoswans: Analyzing fat hatred, weight loss surgery, and compulsory biomedicalized aesthetics in America. *International Journal of Feminist Approaches to Bioethics* **4** (1):188–220.

Morrill, Calvin, K. Tyson, L.B. Edelman, and **R. Arum**. 2010. Legal mobilization in schools: The paradox of rights and race among youth. *Law and Society Review* **44** (3–4):651–94.

Morris, Edward. 2007. "Ladies" or "Loudies"? Perceptions and experiences of Black girls in classrooms. *Youth and Society* **38** (4): 490–515.

Morris, Lisa S. and Richard M. Schultz. 1993. Medication compliance: The patient's perspective. *Clinical Therapeutics: The International Peer-Reviewed Journal of Drug Therapy* **15** (3):593–606.

Morton, Jennifer. 2010. Norms of rationality, epistemic injustice, discounting knowers: Toward an ecological theory of the norms of practical deliberation. *European Journal of Philosophy* **19** (4):561–84.

Murdoch, Iris. 1970. *The sovereignty of good.* London and New York: Routledge.

Murray, C. J., and A.D. Lopez. 1996. *The global burden of disease: A comprehensive assessment of mortality and disability from diseases, injuries, and risk factors in 1990 and projected to 2020.* Cambridge, MA: Harvard School of Public Health.

Nelson, Hilde Lindemann. 2001. *Damaged identities, narrative repair.* Ithaca, NY: Cornell University Press.

Nelson, Lynn Hankinson. 1993. Epistemological communities. In *Feminist epistemologies*, eds. L. Alcoff and E. Potter, 121–60. New York: Routledge.

Neumann, Craig, Robert Hare, and Peter Johansson. 2012. The psychopathy checklist-revised (PCL-R), low anxiety, and fearlessness: A structural equation modeling analysis. *Personality Disorders: Theory, Research, and Treatment* **4** (2):129–37.

Ngoh, Lucy. 2009. Health literacy: A barrier to pharmacist–patient communication and medication adherence. *Journal of the American Pharmacists Association* **49** (5):e132–e149.

Nickerson, R. S. 1998. Confirmation bias: A ubiquitous phenomenon in many guises. *Review of General Psychology 2* (2):175–220.

Nissim-Sabat, Marilyn. 2013. Race and gender in philosophy of psychiatry: Science, relativism, and phenomenology. In *The Oxford handbook of philosophy and psychiatry*, ed. K.W.M. Fulford, M. Davies, G. Graham, R. Gipps, J. Sadler, T. Thornton, and G. Stanghellini, 139–58. Oxford: Oxford University Press.

Noddings, Nel. 1991. *Women and evil.* Berkeley: University of California Press.

Nussbaum, Martha. 1992. Human functioning and social justice: In defense of Aristotelian essentialism. *Political Theory* **20** (2):202–46.

Nussbaum, Martha. 1999. Judging other cultures: The case of genital mutilation. In *Sex and social justice.* Oxford: Oxford University Press.

Nussbaum, Martha. 2000. *Women and human development: The capabilities approach.* Cambridge, MA: Cambridge University Press.

Nussbaum, Martha. 2003. *Upheavals of thought: The intelligence of emotions.* Cambridge, MA: Cambridge University Press.

Nussbaum, Martha. 2006. *Frontiers of justice: Disability, nationality, species membership.* Cambridge, MA: Harvard University Press.

Oglaff, James. 2006. Psychopathy/antisocial personality disorder conundrum. *The Australian and New Zealand Journal of Psychiatry* **40** (6–7):519–28.

Olfson, Mark, David Mechanic, Stephen Hansell, Carol Boyer, et al. 2000. Predicting medication noncompliance after hospital discharge among patients with schizophrenia. *Psychiatric Services*, **51** (2):216–22.

Olson, Parmy. 2012. *We are anonymous: Inside the hacker world of LulzSec, Anonymous, and the global cyber insurgency.* New York: Little, Brown, and Company.

O'Neill, Onora. 1996. *Towards justice and virtue: A constructive account of practical reasoning.* Cambridge, MA: Cambridge University Press.

Ozment, Steven. 1996. *The bürgermeister's daughter: Scandal in a sixteenth-century German town.* New York: St. Martin's Press.

Pachter, Lee, and Cynthia García Coll. 2009. Racism and child health: A review of the literature and future directions. *Journal of Developmental and Behavioral Pediatrics* **30** (3):255–63.

Papadopoulos, F.C., A. Ekbom, L. Brandt, and L. Ekselius. 2009. Excess mortality, causes of death and prognostic factors in anorexia nervosa. *The British Journal of Psychiatry* **194** (1):10–17.

Pelaccia, Thierry, Jacques Tardif, Emmanuel Triby, and Bernard Charlin. 2011. An analysis of clinical reasoning through a recent and comprehensive approach: the dual-process theory. *Medical Education Online* 2011; **16**. Available at http://www.ncbi.nlm.nih.gov/pmc/articles/PMC3060310/nlm.nih.gov/pmc/articles/PMC3060310/.

Pervin, Lawrence. 1994. A critical analysis of current trait theory. *Psychological Inquiry* **5** (2):103–13.

Peterson, Thomas. 2014. Being worse off: But in comparison with what? The baseline problem of harm and the harm principle. *Res Publica* **20** (2):199–214.

Plato. 1974. *The republic.* trans. G.M.A. Grube. Indianapolis: Hackett Pub. Co.

Podell, David, and Leslie Soodak.1993. Teacher efficacy and bias in special education referrals. *Journal of Educational Research* **86** (4):247–53.

Pogge, Thomas. 1999. Human flourishing and universal justice. *Social Philosophy and Policy* **16** (1):333–61.

Porter, Doug. 2015. Colonization and psychiatry. *Journal of Ethics and Mental Health.* Available at http://www.jemh.ca/issues/open/documents/JEMH_Open-Volume_Article_Theme%20_Colonization_Colonization_June2015.pdf. Last accessed: December 20, 2015.

Potter, Nancy Nyquist. 2000. Giving uptake. *Social Theory and Practice* **26** (3):479–508.

Potter, Nancy Nyquist. 2001. Is refusing to forgive a vice? In *Feminists doing ethics*, ed. Peggy DesAutels and Joanne Waugh, 135–50. Lanham, MD: Rowman-Littlefield.

Potter, Nancy Nyquist. 2002. *How can I be trusted? A virtue theory of trustworthiness.* Lanham, MD: Rowman-Littlefield.

Potter, Nancy Nyquist. 2003. Moral tourists and world-travelers: Some epistemological considerations for understanding patients' worlds. *Philosophy, Psychiatry, and Psychology* **10** (3):209–23.

Potter, Nancy Nyquist. 2006. What is manipulative behavior, anyway? *Journal of Personality Disorders* **20** (2):139–56.

Potter, Nancy Nyquist. 2009. *Mapping the edges and the in-between: A critical analysis of borderline personality disorder.* Oxford: Oxford University Press.

Potter, Nancy Nyquist. 2013. Feminist psychiatric ethics in the 21st century and the social context of suffering. In *Oxford handbook of psychiatric ethics*, eds. K.W.M. Fulford, Martin Davies, Richard Gipps, George Graham, John Sadler, Giovanni Stanghellini, and Tim Thornton, 293–306. Oxford: Oxford University Press.

Potter, Nancy Nyquist. 2014. "Oppositional Defiant Disorder: Cultural factors that influence interpretations of defiant behavior and their social and scientific consequences" in *Classifying psychopathology: Mental kinds and natural kinds*, ed. H. Kincaid and J. Sullivan, 175–193. MIT Press.

Potter, Nancy Nyquist. 2015. Defiance, epistemologies of ignorance, and giving uptake properly in psychiatry. In *Diagnostic controversies: Cultural perspectives on competing knowledge in health care*, eds. Carolyn Smith-Morris. New York: Routledge.

Prinz, Jesse. 2007. *The emotional construction of morals*. Oxford: Oxford University Press.

Putallaz, Martha, and **Karen Bierman**, eds. 2004. *Aggression, antisocial behavior, and violence among girls: A developmental perspective*. New York: Guilford Press.

Radden, Jennifer, and **John Sadler**. 2010. *The virtuous psychiatrist: Character ethics in psychiatric practice*. Oxford: Oxford University Press.

Rasmussun, Douglas. 1999. Human flourishing and the appeal to human nature. *Social Philosophy and Policy* **16** (1):1–43

Reading, Anthony. 2004. *Hope and despair: How perceptions of the future shape human behavior*. Baltimore, MD: The John Hopkins University Press.

Reay, Diane. 2001. "Spice girls", "nice girls", "girlies", and "tomboys": Gender discourses, girls' cultures, and femininities in the primary classroom. *Gender and Education* **13** (2):153–66.

Reich, James. 2007. State and trait in personality disorders. *Annals of Clinical Psychiatry* **19** (1):37–44.

Reiland, Rachel. 2004. *Get me out of here: My recovery from borderline personality disorder*. Center City, MN: Hazelden Foundation.

Rich, Adrienne. 1978. Cartographies of silence. In *The dream of a common language*, 16–20. New York: Norton and Co.

Rich, Motoko. 2014. School data finds pattern of inequality along racial lines. *New York Times*, March 3, 2014.

Rieger, Elizabeth, S.W. Touyz, T. Swain, and **P.J. Beumont**. 2001. Cross-cultural research on Anorexia Nervosa: Assumptions regarding the role of body weight. *International Journal of Eating Disorders* **29** (2):205–15.

Riley, D. 1997. *The defiant child: A parent's guide to oppositional defiant disorder*. Lanham, MD: Taylor Trade Publishing.

Robb, Adelaide S., T.J. Silber, J.K. Orrell-Valente, A. Valadez-Meltzer, et al. 2002. Supplemental nocturnal nasogastric refeeding for better short-term outcome in hospitalized adolescent girls with Anorexia Nervosa. *American Journal of Psychiatry* **159** (8):1347–53.

Rorty, Amelie Oksenberg. 2004. The improvisatory dramas of deliberation. In *Setting the moral compass: Essays by women philosophers*, ed. Cheshire Calhoun, 275–87. Oxford: Oxford University Press.

Rosling, Agneta M., P. Sparen, C. Norring, and **A.L. von Knorring**. 2011. Mortality of eating disorders: A follow-up study of treatment in a specialist unit 1974–2000. *International Journal of Eating Disorders* **44** (4):304–10.

Sadler, John. 2005. *Values and psychiatric diagnosis*. Oxford: Oxford University Press.

Sadler, John. 2013a. Vice and mental disorders. In *Oxford handbook of psychiatric ethics*, eds. K.W.M. Fulford, Martin Davies, Richard Gipps, George Graham, John Sadler, Giovanni Stanghellini, and Tim Thornton, 451–79. Oxford: Oxford University Press.

Sadler, John. 2013b. Considering the economy of DSM alternatives. In *Making the DSM-5: Concepts and Controversies*, eds. Joel Paris and James Phillips, 21–38. New York: Springer.

Sadler, John. 2014. Conduct disorder as a vice-laden diagnostic concept. In *Child and adolescent psychiatry: Philosophical perspectives*, eds. Christian Perring and Lloyd Wellls, 166–81. Oxford: Oxford University Press.

Sadler, J.Z., F. Jotterand, S.C. Lee, and **S. Inrig.** 2009. Can medicalization be good? Situating medicalization within bioethics. *Theoretical Medicine and Bioethics* **30** (6):411–25.

Saks, Elyn. 2002. *Refusing care: Forced treatment and the rights of the mentally ill.* Chicago: University of Chicago Press.

Saks, Elyn. 2007. *The center cannot hold: My journey through madness.* New York: Hyperion.

Schonsheck, Jonathan. 2004. Rudeness, rasp, and repudiation. In *Civility and its discontents: Essays on civic virtue, toleration, and cultural fragmentation*, ed. C. T. Sistare, 169–85. Lawrence, Kansas: University of Kansas Press.

Schore, Allan. 2002. Advances in neuropsychoanalysis, attachment theory, and trauma research: Implications for self psychology. *Psychoanalytic Inquiry* **22** (3): 433–84.

Schore, Allan. 2009. Relational trauma and the developing right brain: An interface of psychoanalytic self psychology and neuroscience. *Annals of the New York Academy of Sciences* **1159** (1):189–203.

Scuglik, Deborah, R.D. Alarcon, A.C. Lapeyre III, M.D. Williams, et al. 2007. When the poetry no longer rhymes: Mental health issues among Somali immigrants in the USA. *Transcultural Psychiatry* **44** (4):581–95.

Scull, Andrew. 1983. The domestication of madness. *Medical History* **27** (3):233–48.

Seal, Mark. 2012. *The man in the Rockefeller suit: The astonishing rise and spectacular fall of a serial imposter.* New York: Penguin Group.

Sen, Amartya. 1985. *Commodities and capabilities.* North-Holland.

Shelton, Deborah. 2004. Experiences of detained young offenders in need of mental health care. *Journal of Nursing Scholarship* **36** (2):129–33.

Sherman, Nancy. 1989. *The fabric of character: Aristotle's theory of virtue.* Oxford: Clarendon Press.

Shorter, Edward. 1998. *A history of psychiatry: From the era of the asylum to the age of Prozac.* Indianapolis, IN: Wiley.

Simpson, K.J. 2002. Anorexia nervosa and culture. *Journal of Psychiatric and Mental Health Nursing* **9** (1):65–71.

Sittenfeld, Curtis. 2001. Your life as a girl. In *Listen up! Voices from the next feminist generation*, ed. Barbara Findlen, 3–10. Emeryville, CA: Seal Press.

Skeem, Jennifer, and **David Cook.** 2010. Is criminal behavior a central component of psychopathy? Conceptual directions for resolving the debate. *Psychological Assessment* **22** (2):433–45.

Skeem, Jennifer, John Edens, Jacqueline Camp, and **Lori Colwell.** 2004. Are there ethnic differences in levels of psychopathy? A meta-analysis. *Law and Human Behavior* **28** (5):505–27.

Slater, Lauren. 1996. *Welcome to my country.* New York: Random House.

Solomon, Andrew. 2002. *Noonday demon: An atlas of depression.* New York: Simon & Schuster.

Sorabji, Richard. 1980. Aristotle on the role of intellect in virtue. In: *Essays on Aristotle's ethics*, ed. A. Rorty, 201–19. Berkeley and Los Angeles: University of California Press.

Stewart, Douglas and Joseph DeMarco. 2010. Rational noncompliance with prescribed medical treatment. *Kennedy Institute of Ethics Journal* **20** (3):277–90.

Sullivan, E.A., C.S. Abramowitz, M. Lopez, et al. 2006. Reliability and construct validity of the psychopathy checklist—revised for Latino, European American, and African American male inmates. *Psychological Assessment* **18** (4):382–92.

Swetz, Keith M., Abdi A. Jama, Onelis Quirindongo-Cedeno, and Lena Hatchett. 2011 Meeting the needs of Somali patients at the end of life. *Minnesota Medicine* **94** (12):43–6.

Szasz, Thomas. 2000. Second commentary on Aristotle's function argument. *Philosophy, psychiatry and psychology* **7** (1):3–17.

Tauber, Alfred. 2007. Balancing medicine's moral ledger: Realigning trust and responsibility. In *Responsibilty*. Ed. B. Darling-Smith, 129–48. Lanham, MD: Rowman & Littlefield Publishers, Inc.

Taylor, Barbara. 2015. *The last asylum: A memoir of madness in our times.* Chicago: University of Chicago Press.

Tec, Nechama. 2009. *Defiance.* Oxford: Oxford University Press.

Tessman, Lisa. 2005. *Burdened virtues: Virtue ethics for liberatory struggles.* Oxford: Oxford University Press.

Tessman, Lisa. 2009. Feminist eudaimonism: Eudaimonism as non-ideal theory. In *Feminist ethics and social and political philosophy: Theorizing the non-ideal*, ed. L. Tessman, 47–58. New York: Springer.

Tessman, Lisa. 2015. *Moral failure: On the impossible demands of morality.* Oxford: Oxford University Press.

Thorton, Tim. 2000. Mental illness and reductionism: Can functions be naturalized? *Philosophy, Psychiatry, and Psychology* **7** (1): 67–77.

Tse, Samson, Jessica Tang, and Alice Kan Dip Cert. 2015. Patient involvement in mental health care: Culture, communication, and caution. *Health Expectations* **18** (1): 3–7.

U.S. Department of Education. 2014. Expansive survey of America's public schools reveals troubling racial disparities: Lack of access to pre-School, greater suspensions cited. March 21, 2014. http://www.ed.gov/news/press-releases/expansive-survey-americas-public-schools-reveals-troubling-racial-disparities. Last accessed January 20, 2015.

U.S. Department of Education Office for Civil Rights. 2014. Civil rights data collection data snapshot: School Discipline. http://ocrdata.ed.gov/Downloads/CRDC-School-Discipline-Snapshot.pdf. Accessed June 25, 2015.

Ussher, Jane. 2011. *The madness of women: Myth and experience.* London and New York: Routledge.

Vuckovich, Paula. 2010. Compliance versus adherence in serious and persistent mental illness. *Nursing Ethics* **17** (1):77–85.

Walker, Margaret Urban. 2007. *Moral understandings: A feminist study in ethics*, 2nd edn. Oxford: Oxford University Press.

Waller, R., F. Gardner, and L. W. Hyde. 2013. What are the associations between parenting, callous-unemotional traits, and antisocial behavior in youth? A systematic review of evidence. *Clinical Psychology Review* **33** (4):593–608.

Watters, Ethan. 2010. *Crazy like us: The globalization of the American psyche.* New York: Free Press.

Western, B. 2006. *Punishment and inequality in America.* New York: Russell Sage Foundation.

Williams, Bernard. 1973. A critique of utilitarianism. In *Utilitarianism: For and against,* J.J.C. Smart and B. Williams, 77–150. Cambridge, Mass: Cambridge University Press.

Wissink, L., R. Jones-Webb, D. Dubois, B. Krinke, et al. 2005. Improving health care provisions to Somali refugee women. *Minnesota Medicine* **88** (2):36–40.

Wittgenstein, Ludwig. 2009. *Philosophical investigations,* 4th edn., trans. G.E.M. Anscombe, eds. P.M.S. Hacker and J. Schulte. Chichester: Wiley-Blackwell.

Woods, Ruth. 2013. *Children's moral lives: An ethnographic and psychological approach.* Malden, MA: John Wiley & Sons, Ltd.

Woolfolk, Robert, and Dominic Murphy. 2004. Axiological foundations of psychotherapy. *Journal of Psychotherapy Integration* **14** (2):168–91.

World Health Organization. 2003. *Adherence to long-term therapies: Evidence for action,* ed. Eduardo Sabaté. Geneva, Switzerland: World Health Organization.

Young, Iris Marion. 2011. *Justice and the politics of difference.* Princeton, NJ: Princeton University Press.

Zahn-Waxler, C., R. J. Ianotti, M.E. Cummings, and S. Denham. 1990. Antecedents of problem behaviors in children of depressed mothers. *Development and Psychopathology* **2** (3):271–91.

Index

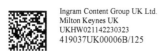